In The Morning Came The Light

Abbey Spinelli

HARVEST VALE BOOKS
AUSTRALIA

Copyright © 2025 by Abbey Spinelli

All rights reserved. No part of this publication may be reproduced, distributed or transmitted in any form or by any means, without prior written permission.

Harvest Vale Books
Australia

Unless otherwise noted, Scripture taken from the Holy Bible, New International Version ® Copyright © 1973, 1978, 1984 by International Bible Society. Used by permission of Zondervan Publishing House. All rights reserved.

Scripture quotation marked CEV is taken from the Contemporary English Version (CEV) Copyright © 1995 by American Bible Society.

Book Layout © 2017 BookDesignTemplates.com

In The Morning Came The Light / Abbey Spinelli -- 1st ed.
ISBN 9780646722399

In The Morning Came The Light

"This is a deeply personal story set in a unique time in history. Abbey recounts her journey in vivid detail battling and recovering from life threatening illness in the intensive care unit. Beyond the accurate and detailed ICU experiences, this book is a reminder that health care is as much about providing hope and reassurance as it is about medicines and machines."
> Professor Ed Litton - Intensive Care Specialist and Director of ICU Research at Fiona Stanley Hospital, Perth, Western Australia.

"In this moving, courageous account, Abbey gives voice to the silence of sedation, the unseen sacrifices of family, and the slow work of healing beyond the ICU walls. Her story of surviving ECMO during Covid isolation is not only extraordinary, but beautifully told – raw, honest and full of grace. This is a book that reminds us that hope is not naïve, love is not optional and recovery is never just physical. It is a vital addition to the growing chorus of patients helping us all to understand medicine more clearly – and more humanely."
> Dr Matt Morgan - Intensive Care Consultant at University Hospital of Wales and author of 'A Second Act'.

"Abbey's story reminds us that tragedy can strike suddenly. Yet her testimony of the power of prayer, the unity of people in faith and the rediscovering of meaning after life-changing trauma points to the faithfulness of God in bringing purpose out of the pain."
> Timothy A. van Aarde - author of 'Discover Your Purpose in the Plan of God'.

For Matt, Jesaia and Coby.
And for my parents Struan and Jill.
This book is my "I love you."

To those who loved us during that time with prayer,
compassion, acts of kindness, presence and fierce faith.
With all my heart, thank you.

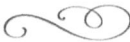

The first part of this book was written with the help of
journals faithfully kept by my
husband Matthew (Matt) and mother Jill while
I was in hospital.

I'm so very thankful for them.

You intended to harm me, but God intended it for good, to accomplish what is now being done.

(Genesis 50:20)

CONTENTS

FOREWORD 11
PROLOGUE 17
CHAPTER ONE 21
CHAPTER TWO 31
CHAPTER THREE 35
CHAPTER FOUR 43
CHAPTER FIVE 47
CHAPTER SIX 55
CHAPTER SEVEN 59
CHAPTER EIGHT 63
CHAPTER NINE 69
CHAPTER TEN 73
CHAPTER ELEVEN 81
CHAPTER TWELVE 87
CHAPTER THIRTEEN 97
CHAPTER FOURTEEN 107
CHAPTER FIFTEEN 115
CHAPTER SIXTEEN 121
CHAPTER SEVENTEEN 129

CHAPTER EIGHTEEN 135
CHAPTER NINETEEN 141
CHAPTER TWENTY.. 151
CHAPTER TWENTY ONE... 157
CHAPTER TWENTY TWO 161
CHAPTER TWENTY THREE 169
CHAPTER TWENTY FOUR... 181
CHAPTER TWENTY FIVE 193
CHAPTER TWENTY SIX... 203
CHAPTER TWENTY SEVEN... 209

Foreword

As one whose professional craft involves being constantly and deeply immersed in the unique space that is critical care medicine, it is a rare gift to be privileged to bear witness to the inspiring testimony that Abbey relates - and a powerful reminder of what often motivates healthcare providers in striving to contribute to enabling such remarkable outcomes. It has been a humbling and daunting prospect to honour the extraordinary story Abbey has recounted in these pages, as someone who shared a small part in her journey. Near the end of her book Abbey relates her trepidation at public speaking, and finds strength and encouragement in the biblical recount of Moses' response to God's provision. Penning these words of foreword to introduce Abbey's narrative fills me with similar disquiet.

Abbey's detailed and intimate portrayal of the trials and tribulations of the often harrowing, precarious state of life in the intensive care unit vividly captures the human costs and aftermath of such an experience. Lifting the veil on so many facets of the exceptional practices within ICU is a welcome addition to the memoirs of critical illness, particularly in the context of the unchartered territory of covid-era restrictions and the many and varying ripples of the first pandemic in nearly a century. Abbey's experience is indeed unique within Western Australia, as the only recipient of ECMO life support for Covid during the pandemic phase – and most exceptionally for requiring support for cardiogenic shock, rather than unsupportable respiratory failure. This seeming notoriety clearly had unsettling consequences for Abbey as she re-assimilated back into her community. The extraordinary form of life support that Abbey required – ECMO – remains an infrequently deployed form of support, limited to the small number of otherwise unsupportable heart and/or lung failure patients on maximal organ-failure supports, and has become paradigm-changing in restoring previously irretrievable clinical situations to remarkable recoveries in some cases. However, it is also a highly invasive technique with considerable risks associated with deploying it – as Abbey graphically describes. Fortunately, in Abbey's case this proceeded remarkably smoothly – though her retelling of the many after-effects is a reminder of the long road to recovery even in the most positive of outcomes. ECMO is a high-cost, high-profile frontier-pushing technology that has seen dramatic growth in use in recent years. Raising awareness of the remarkable recoveries that can be engendered with its skilled deployment is to be applauded, and all of us that are involved in the extraordinary endeavours of meticulously implementing ECMO are keen to support more awareness of these outcomes.

Abbey's experiences also provide insight into another frequently overlooked aspect of critical illness – the often dark, terrifying journey of mental torment that can be pervasive and all-consuming for a substantial proportion of patients, both during the life-threatening acute phase and for prolonged periods in the aftermath. These graphic and destabilising symptoms can return seemingly inexplicably to haunt sufferers long into the future. While the underlying critical illness and its consequences are usually the primary contributors to these distressing symptoms, all too often the medications we utilise to treat the primary disease or, as in Abbey's case, provide a safe medically induced coma, as well as the often-unavoidable disturbance of sleep patterns, exacerbate the acute phase of a distorted perception of reality experienced by the patient. Unfortunately this often lays the foundation for longer-term distressing psychological symptoms, such as post-traumatic stress disorder. In sharing her story, Abbey provides a reassuring account of the journey to accommodate these distressing interjections in life after critical illness.

The ramifications of Covid had profound impacts on the experience of medical care for patients such as Abbey and their immediate family members, as well as the many healthcare providers working under exceptionally challenging circumstances. The sense of emotional distress for many patients left scars that persisted long after the acute phase of recovery. Indeed Abbey's recount of her experience lays bare the sense of disconnection and alienation as a result, while her family members' journals vividly capture the emotional turmoil of the situation. The unique difficulties of this time also contributed to healthcare provider burnout, and substantial staff exodus – often of our most experienced team members. Abbey's narrative is also a reminder of the many layers of moral hazard and ethical dilemmas that were prominent at the time, such as constraints around patient visiting policies.

Perhaps the most illuminating and inspiring aspect of Abbey's journey is her faith and its impact on her approach to the psychological aftermath of her harrowing journey. It is impossible not to be moved and affected by her frequent reference to the biblical foundation of her faith as a refuge and sense of strength. The depth and breadth of a vibrant Christian community reaching out with love, prayer and practical help to support Abbey and her family during that time is a wonderful testament to the altruistic sense of connection in the faith community they are a part of.

It has been a privilege to play a small part in Abbey's journey, and awe-inspiring to see the witness she has been in so many environments since her experience with life-threatening illness. I commend her testimony to all those with a curiosity about the journey through critical illness and the deeply personal path to recovery.

Dr Christopher Allen
Senior ICU Intensivist and ECMO Lead
Fiona Stanley Hospital, Perth, Western Australia

Prologue

Sunday 8th March 2020
Three days before the world as we knew it officially imploded. Half an hour earlier, the magical moment had been one of innocence and ignorant bliss. My husband Matt and I had been sitting in the snow-covered town square of Tromso, Norway – far into the Arctic Circle, and almost fourteen thousand kilometres from our home on the opposite side of the globe in sun-drenched Western Australia. With our gloved hands wrapped around mugs of hot chocolate, we couldn't stop grinning as we watched our two young sons working together to build a fort in the thick snow nearby, stopping regularly to pelt increasingly larger snowballs at each other. This had been a trip five long years in the making, planning and saving, beginning with a photograph in a book and a dream to see the Northern Lights. As time marched on and our dreams of an Arctic adventure became closer to reality, our excitement grew, as did an almost sense of disbelief – was our half-decade of saving and planning actually, finally going to turn into real-life snow, reindeers, huskies and the magical Northern Lights?

In the weeks before our trip there'd been talk and increasing media coverage of a virus – now known as COVID-19 – that was picking up pace in its spread across the globe, but it didn't seem connected to the far reaches of the Arctic Circle. Yet now, standing in front of the hut serving hot drinks in that magical Tromso town square, ready to buy a second hot chocolate in a bid to stretch out the glorious afternoon, the woman serving our drinks uttered the words that brought instant unease to the moment, "Did you hear that covid has hit Tromso? Hotels are locking down."

Within twenty-four hours the small Arctic city that had captivated us with its breathtaking scenery began to close down rapidly, and the following days would become an increasing whirlwind of confusion, phone calls to and from Australia, waiting, tears, panic and frantic decision-making. Our family of four would fly from Tromso to the Norwegian capital, Oslo, where we sat anxiously in our rented apartment, watching through the window as the country's Prime Minister got out of her car on the pavement below and walked into Parliament House to announce the decision to lock down the nation.

Our long-awaited Arctic adventure was over before it had barely begun.

Devastated, we flew out of a chaotic Oslo Airport the next day, with security guards wearing PPE yelling at frantic travellers to "Keep a safe distance!" and "Stand back!", and both adults and children alike crying while waiting for flights – tears of fear, confusion and dawning realisation. Our family arrived in London, where we were greeted with casual friendliness in customs, the officer more interested in how we'd managed to release our boys from Australian schooling during the term rather than the concern of potential coronavirus. So we naively decided we could transfer our dream trip to England, stay awhile there. We spent one abnormally quiet and blue-skied London day travelling on the almost-empty Tube, visiting a near-deserted Museum of Natural History (which, as it would turn out, would close the very next day for more than a year), and watching the London Eye turn its repeated circle, bereft of its usual excited tourists. And then the Australian Government ordered us home, slamming shut the nation's borders, along with our last-ditch attempt to salvage something – anything – of our family adventure. Matt spent a frenzied day at Heathrow Airport, battling the crowds of travellers from around the world desperately trying to achieve the same outcome – securing a flight to take us all home. Bitterly disappointed tears marked the journey from London to Doha, where we spent a night wandering the eerily hushed airport, peering into the darkened windows of shops that were now firmly closed in the onset of the pandemic. After another tear-filled and now vomit-plagued flight – with our exhausted eldest son gripped by relentless motion sickness for the entire eleven hour journey home – we finally made it back to Australia, alongside the German backpacker who asked for our translating help in customs at Perth Airport, telling us he was "disappearing into the bush for as long as this virus thing hangs around". We entered into two weeks of mandatory home quarantine, spending Matt's birthday watching *The Lion King* movie in our loungeroom, rather than the stage show we'd had tickets for in London's West End. We began what would become an eight month battle with our travel insurance company to redeem the expenses of our broken trip. And we questioned, over and over, how an adventure of a lifetime that was five years in the making could have fallen exactly at this time – naïve, as everyone was, as to how long 'this time' would actually go on for.

Little did we know 'this virus thing' had much more in store for our family. Panic, tears, phone calls, PPE and quarantine would repeat themselves. But this time, instead of losing a holiday, I would almost lose my life.

Chapter One

Friday 8th April 2022
It was the feeling of being pinned down, unable to move, that first hit me. Then the pain that seemed to be coursing through my veins, and a sickness that was unlike anything I'd ever felt, all-consuming and overwhelming. Everything was white, disorienting and out of focus. I must be dying, I decided – the irony of which I would later understand. Just as I was begging death to come quickly, to release me from this agonising state, a space creature appeared at my side. She was, in reality, a nurse, but in my world of delirium and confusion there was nothing human to grasp about the full-body PPE she was wearing – the cap, goggles, mask, gown, gloves and face visor refused to reveal any comforting features. The voice was human though. She gently greeted me, explaining that I was now awake, that I'd been "very, very sick". I couldn't understand what she was telling me, didn't recognize anything or anyone that could make sense of where I was. "You have covid", she said, and suddenly my brain latched onto a flash of memory – 'covid'. That's right, I'd had covid. My husband had had covid. My boys had had covid. I had a husband and children. I had a family – I

knew that much! And then the sickness took hold again, and it became too hard to think, to remember. I needed to escape the bed that was pinning me to my pain, but I was trapped by tubes, everywhere. I wanted someone to do something – anything – to take away the overpowering monster of sickness. And then the panic set in.

Eight days earlier… Thursday 31st March 2022
So much had changed in the past week. The previous Wednesday we'd been celebrating Matt's forty-first birthday by taking our kayaks and a picnic lunch to Little Rock, a beautifully peaceful and scenic spot on the Collie River around half an hour from home. The sun was shining, the water was cool and calm, and the temperature was perfect for paddling and a post-lunch snooze. And yet I hadn't been able to relax my unsettled mind that day. Looking back I don't believe it was intuition – mercifully, I had no idea of what was to come. Now, a little over a week later, all four of us – Matt and myself, and our two boys, twelve-year-old Jesaia and nine-year-old Coby – had contracted covid. As March moved into April, the timing was on the cusp of the peak of the pandemic in Western Australia. After two years and counting of a range of government restrictions, WA's hard border had been lifted just three weeks before, allowing for the early beginnings of both interstate and overseas travel for the first time

since March 2020. With covid case numbers now rising rapidly in WA, it was an environment of heightened emotion, anxiety and uncertainty in the community, with many people feeling the painful effects of social and family divisions, separation and loneliness. And in the thick of this our family of four had gone down one after the other with the virus, like proverbial dominoes. Looking on the positive side, we were relieved that our requisite period of close-contact home isolation could be done in one go, all together. Matt – the last of the four to test positive – was just at the start of his illness, while our boys were already starting to feel better. We all agreed the burning, ripping sore throat was the worst. And now it was Thursday evening, nearing the end of the day in which I'd actually started to see a slight improvement in my covid symptoms. I was preparing my son's bed for sleep when it hit me – an overwhelming and alarming weakness, as though every last bit of strength and energy had been sucked from my body. An increasing heaviness in my legs forced me to collapse onto the bed, unable to even contemplate having the strength to get up again. And that's where I stayed until the middle of the night, when I got out of my son's bed and walked across the house to my bedroom, my legs feeling as though they were made of cement, each step a distressing effort to make in my severe weakness. I found Matt awake in bed, despite the early hour of 3am, his fiery sore throat making it impossible for him to sleep. "Something is very wrong" I told him, struggling to find the strength to stay upright or even talk. After telling my husband about the concrete legs, the heaviness in walking, the overwhelming weakness and the increasing shakiness, Matt made a call first to my parents (as children often do, no matter how grown up we are), and then to a tele-health service for advice on what to do. Are these normal symptoms for covid? Should we go to a hospital? Wait to speak to a GP? "We're not sure without being able to see you... possibly hold off on the hospital trip... definitely get in contact with your doctor as soon as you can", came the reply. We waited on the living room couch, watching the minutes on the clock and the strength in my body slowly slip away, until our tiny corner of the world started opening up for the day, and Matt could call our family GP. "Unfortunately the doctor doesn't have an available appointment until 4pm today... would you like us to book Abbey in for a tele-appointment then?" A brief discussion and the decision was to made to try to find another doctor with an earlier appointment – a course of action that would see Matt driving me to Bunbury Hospital a few short hours later, my father having to sit in his car on our driveway to keep watch over our two boys who were inside the house, mostly recovered in their symptoms but still testing positive to covid.

I will take a moment here to say that I had no memory at all of any of this – the heaviness, the collapsing on the bed, the phone calls, the later trip to Bunbury Hospital – until weeks and even months later, when memories would start to return, some crashing into my mind without warning, others slowly filtering in during conversation with others.

But now, the doctor on the phone was telling Matt to take me to Bunbury Hospital. It would be faster for Matt to take me himself, the doctor said, rather than wait for a covid-specialty ambulance. The doctor would call ahead to the hospital, let them know to have someone waiting for me. Matt would be allowed out of quarantine to drive me, the GP said, but would need to stay with the car at the hospital. One memory that would return weeks later was trying to shower before heading to the hospital, now so overcome with weakness that I couldn't even raise my hands to rinse my hair or turn off the taps. Laying on our bed afterwards, I was vaguely aware of Matt darting around the room in panic, trying to pack a bag with supplies for a trip to hospital he thought might be for a night, but would turn out to be so much more. Months later, another flicker of memory would push its way to the surface, when our son Coby shared with me how I'd lain on the couch in our lounge room, barely coherent, as he tried to stir me to go to the hospital with Matt. And then, with no recollection of the drive there, we were at Bunbury Hospital, Matt pulling into the drop-off bay and running around to my car door to help me out. What came towards us then, one of whom was pushing a wheelchair, were two aliens, the first of many I'd come across over the coming weeks. Faces obscured by goggles, white surgical masks and clear plastic face shields, their bodies covered in blue space suits, the aliens – in actual fact, hospital staff – called out to Matt to stay where he was, as they eased me into the wheelchair and placed a shield over my own masked face. And then the aliens swiftly wheeled me into the hospital, with Matt left standing alone by the car, confused and desperately helpless.

Matt's journal – Friday 1st April, afternoon
It was the most horrible feeling leaving you at the entrance to ED, being wheelchaired away by two people in full PPE. You looked so frightened in your mask and face shield. I couldn't even give you a proper hug or kiss before you left.

Months later, through many emotion-filled conversations with Matt, my parents and doctors, I'd wade through the puzzle pieces of what happened next, sometimes bringing on a fleeting snippet of memory that my brain would struggle to grasp hold of. Being taken into an isolation room within the hospital's emergency department to wait… texting an increasingly anxious Matt back at home with the desperate message *"I feel as though I'm going to faint"*… being moved into the intensive care unit, where it became increasingly apparent the doctors were dealing not with a respiratory issue (the initial thought, given I had covid), but with a heart in serious trouble. Blood tests were taken and results quickly returned. Troponin – which is a protein that's released into the blood during heart failure - usually measures at undetectable levels for a healthy heart, and around 40 for a probable heart attack. My results came back at a terrifying 7,000 – later to rise to 13,000 when I'd be medically flown to Perth – indicating severe heart damage. Despite being given the intravenous antiviral medication remdesivir my condition began to deteriorate overnight, and by early the next morning the situation had become seriously dire. The left ventricle of my heart was shutting down, and cardiogenic shock was diagnosed – a life-threatening condition in which the heart has been damaged so extensively that it's unable to pump enough blood to the brain and vital organs. I was going into acute heart failure.

Jill's journal – Friday 1st April, night
You're now in ICU where you've had nausea and spells of unconsciousness. Your dad and I spoke to you over the phone this evening – your speech was slurred and slow, and you had to stop talking after only a short while. You didn't even sound like our Abbey.

Matt's journal – Saturday 2nd April, morning
The ICU doctors in Bunbury Hospital say you're not responding to any of the treatment they're giving you. Your heart is deteriorating, so the decision has been made to fly you to Fiona Stanley Hospital in Perth. An ambulance will take you to Bunbury Airport at around 11am. I've packed some more things for you, which your parents will bring to the hospital, because I'm not allowed to be there.

Heart failure, however, has little regard for plans. An episode of VT (ventricular tachycardia - a fast, abnormal heart rhythm) led to me fainting and doctors placing shock pads on my chest. With my condition rapidly deteriorating, I lost consciousness while medical staff tried to transfer me from my hospital bed to the ambulance trolley. The grave concern that I wouldn't survive the forty-five minute flight to Perth now became very real. After a phone call with doctors at Fiona Stanley Hospital, the decision was made to persist with getting me on the plane – I needed treatment in Perth to have any chance of survival.

Chapter Two

Jill's journal – Saturday 2nd April, afternoon
Your dad and I waited outside the hospital entrance for more than two hours. Different nurses would come out to let us know where to stand, what door they would bring you through to the ambulance, and how close we could be from the ambulance (three metres) to see you. We didn't know the doctors were having enormous trouble taking you a few short corridors of the hospital to the ambulance, because you'd become extremely fragile and unstable, and were at high risk of cardiac arrest. At around 1pm, a nurse suggested we come inside to the ICU family lounge to get something to eat. It was then you were finally transferred to the ambulance and onto the airport, two hours delayed. We were so disappointed to have not been able to see you, but we understood how they couldn't have any distraction or disruption in the difficult and dangerous transfer. An ICU doctor carefully and honestly answered all of our questions and concerns. She explained that you're very unwell, and there was a real risk you wouldn't survive the flight to Perth and then the ambulance transfer to Fiona Stanley Hospital. She told us that a specialist doctor would be with you for the entire journey. We've returned home in shock.

Before my parents arrived home, however, they had to face the incredibly surreal situation of stopping by the supermarket to do a grocery shop for Matt and our boys, who needed food supplies but couldn't go to the shops themselves due to quarantine restrictions. Dad and Mum would later describe moving through the aisles of the supermarket in a foggy haze, unable to comprehend the normal Saturday activity that swirled around them as people went about their shopping completely oblivious to the life or death situation unfolding in my parents' world. The feeling of their disconnect and of concealed pain and grief in that moment was intense. The adage that we never know what's going on in the life of the many strangers we pass in any given day was never more real than in that moment, and it's a reminder that I try hard to live by each day – that the person walking past us in the shops, standing in the queue in front of us, or driving in their car alongside us just might be experiencing the most difficult or painful of situations in their life.

And that day, those strangers in the supermarket fighting back fear, distress and tears were my parents.

At this very time, a powerful and increasingly bold prayer chain was growing, which would rapidly extend to a number of countries around the world, and carry Matt, our boys and my parents through the coming days of desperate uncertainty. At Bunbury Airport, as I was being prepared to be placed on the Royal Flying Doctor Service plane, my condition further deteriorated, and I had another episode of losing consciousness. I would later be told by a cardiologist that the left ventricle of my barely pumping heart was functioning at less than 10 percent during the flight to Perth. This measurement of the percentage of blood leaving the heart each time it squeezes is known as ejection fraction. To put my situation into perspective, a heart functioning at twenty-five percent is classified as severely impaired and indicative of significant heart failure, while an ejection fraction of fifteen percent is usually seen in end-stage or transplant patients. A heart pumping at less than ten percent can easily lead to death – mine was later described by a cardiologist as a medically 'nonfunctional' heart. To fly me over 150 kilometres while treating a heart that was so rapidly deteriorating was incredibly risky, and very challenging for all involved. And so we know with unshakeable confidence and immense gratitude that, alongside the skilled medical staff who cared for me so urgently on that two-hour air and road journey between two hospitals, God was very much present in both ambulances and on the plane, my failing heart being held in the hands of its Creator.

At around 2pm, Matt, Jesaia and Coby would stand outside in our suburban backyard and helplessly watch as a plane flew high in the sky overhead, tracking it as it headed north towards Perth, wondering if their wife and mother was onboard. Coby would climb as high as he possibly could on the tallest frame of his monkey bars, bridging the gap between himself and the plane.

And the prayers of so many carried my family through that desperate flight as well.

Chapter Three

Matt's journal – Saturday 2nd April, evening
You arrived safely at Fiona Stanley Hospital around 4pm, which was a huge relief. A few hours later I had several calls from the ICU consultant, Reena, and things were getting very scary as your condition continued to deteriorate. You had lost consciousness twice, and the medical team started preparing me over the phone that they were getting ready to put you on a life support machine called ECMO.

ECMO. An acronym of four letters we'd never heard of before, which now has a very personal meaning to our family. ECMO – which stands for Extracorporeal Membrane Oxygenation – was described to Matt at the time as being the highest level of life support for the sickest of the sick. Patients needing to be put on ECMO are suffering a life-threatening illness that's led to severe lung or heart failure (in my case, cardiogenic shock). The ECMO machine works as a type of artificial life support, taking over the job of the lungs or, as in my situation, the heart – draining the blood out of the body via tubing, adding oxygen and removing carbon dioxide, and pumping the blood back into the patient.

Only a relatively small number of hospitals in Australia – and only two in WA – are able to provide ECMO life support in their intensive care unit, with highly specialised equipment and staff needed for constant supervision.

Incredible and lifesaving as it is, ECMO is often considered a life support of last resort, when other treatment options aren't working. This is because ECMO support comes with a number of life-threatening risks, including bleeding, kidney failure, bacterial infection, sepsis, stroke and blood clots. Severely reduced blood circulation can also lead to the devastating threat of limb amputation. Considering the patient on ECMO is already seriously unwell, any one of these potential risks can ultimately prove fatal.

For Matt – who'd never even heard of ECMO before – being told these risks was his first introduction to the life-support machine that would soon be attached to his critically ill wife.

Matt's journal – Saturday 2nd April, evening
Reena explained to me that because your condition is so poor, the risks of putting you on the ECMO machine are high, and they haven't made the decision lightly. She told me that your

heart is very weak and not pumping enough blood around your body, and that without the support of ECMO, you won't survive the night. I had no choice but to trust and say yes.

Much later, Matt would share with me that conversation, and the anguish of having those life-threatening risks compassionately but frankly laid out to him over the phone. The nurse explained the harsh reality – given how critically diseased my heart was, there was a more than fifty percent chance I wouldn't survive on the ECMO life support. In panic and tears Matt phoned my parents, who encouraged him to trust in the decision-making of the ECMO team. Literally trapped in our home, 150 kilometres away, not allowed to be by my side, Matt had little other choice. It seemed like the cruelest of situations.

Matt's journal – Saturday 2nd April, evening
I was desperate to talk to you before the doctors took you to theatre. At first Reena said you wouldn't be able to speak to me, and I was distraught that I couldn't talk to you before you went onto the life support. About half an hour later, a nurse called me using your phone, saying you'd be able to talk to me briefly. I was so happy to have that time. We only talked for a few minutes, but I told you how much I missed you, and that I wished I was there with you. I was just so relieved to hear your

voice, which sounded angelic to me, and to be able to tell you that I loved you. Jesaia and Coby spoke to you as well, and told you they loved you too.

I have no memory at all of these final conversations with Matt and our boys before doctors induced my coma and attached the life support. To this day, that remains an incredibly difficult thing to wrap my head around, and the thought that those words shared between us in those precious minutes could have been my last haunted my mind for a long time afterwards.

Jill's journal – Saturday 2nd April, evening
Before putting you on life support, doctors made the decision to perform a risky procedure that involved inserting a tube with a camera attached into your groin, up through the heart, and back through the other groin. They needed to see the extent of the damage to your heart, and whether there were any blockages. Your veins and arteries were clear, but your heart is very inflamed and swollen.

It was another intensely high-risk situation. A medically 'non-functional' heart, a body facing the threat of organ failure from cardiogenic shock, just hours before I was placed into a coma on life support that would last for the next week. Yet again, to know afterwards that this had all been happening around me – to me – without any understanding or memory was very hard to comprehend. However, when I think about the urgency and decision-making that would have driven that moment in the hospital theatre, the overwhelming emotion I feel is gratitude – for the skilled hands of the medical team who were working so carefully under growing pressure, and for the faithful hands of my God who held that swollen and failing heart in His loving protection.

Matt's journal – Saturday 2nd April, night
I read Dr Seuss' 'Oh, the Places You'll Go!' to Jesaia and Coby before they went to bed. We chose this book because it's your favourite to read. We cuddled and prayed, and both boys seemed peaceful as they went to sleep.
Just after 10pm, Reena phoned me again to say you were now back in ICU, and were calm and peaceful during the procedure. You are now in an induced coma, with the ECMO machine supporting your heart by pumping your blood.
I wonder how much of this day you will remember? I will always remember this day as the one when I could lose the love of my life.

How much of this day do I remember? Very, very little. Virtually nothing, in fact. It's hard to put into words how strange, how incredibly difficult it is to know that so much happened – to me, to my heart, to my body, to my precious family – on this day which, by the grace of God, could have been my last... and yet *I just don't remember*. Two fleeting memories from that day have come back to me over the months – the first of being pushed on a bed down a corridor (which I now know was Bunbury Hospital, as they worked to transfer me to the waiting ambulance), feeling my eyes roll back in my head as I slipped into darkness, an overwhelming sense of relief that I could escape the all-consuming illness. The second flash of memory from that day was incredibly upsetting, and came much earlier in my post-hospital recovery – a confusing snippet of a picture in my brain that saw me in the ambulance travelling on a Perth freeway to Fiona Stanley Hospital, the doctor treating me as he urgently questioned the driver on how long we had left to go in the journey. Again, darkness consumed me, and I slipped into a memory-less state that would hold me for the next week.

Dad's text message to my phone – Saturday 2nd April, night
We love you SO much our darling Ab, we wish we could be with you now. We will see you soon, our precious girl. We love you. Dad and Mum xoxo

This was the first of many text messages my loving dad sent to my phone while I was on life support, despite knowing that the coma held me in a place that wouldn't allow me to read them. Unable to be by my bedside, he was desperate to connect with me in a tangible way, and determined that I would receive the messages when – not *if* – I woke from the coma. Starting from that first night, he and my mum would also call through every evening to the phone in my ICU room, which the nurse would then place on speaker. Using words of encouragement and strength, and often drawing on the promises of scripture, my parents would talk to me as though they were in the room with me. They would always end the one-sided conversation in prayer, trusting that God would penetrate the words deep into my conscience.

I know with all my healed heart that He lovingly did exactly that.

Chapter Four

Matt's journal – Sunday 3rd April, very early morning
I'm not able to sleep. I've cried a lot. I feel shock and disbelief.
I'm scared and confused.

Most people would expect that being trapped in your home while your wife is placed into a coma on life support 150 kilometres away, unwell yourself, unable to accept visitors and facing a long, dark night ahead, would make for an incredibly lonely space to be in. And yet... Matt will tell you that he truly never felt alone during that first desperate night, or in the nights to come. Scared, confused, in shock – very much so. But never alone in the presence of his Heavenly Father. There were the many messages, including one from a friend at 2am on that first night, as Matt lay wide awake staring at the ceiling, that read, *"I'm awake and I'm praying"*. Matt's message of response in his fear and distress? A bold declaration of trust - *"Our God is mighty to save"*. Matt would later find out that many, many others were also wide awake that night – in kneeled positions by bedsides, pacing hallways, huddled over in lounge chairs - interceding in desperate and bold prayer for my survival. To this day, I have a powerful image in my mind of these hundreds of faithful prayer warriors, in homes around the country, doing battle against death - their weapon of choice being to cry out to the Almighty Healer. Over the months after returning home from hospital, Matt and I would hear countless stories of the ways God moved and challenged people to pray to Him on that first night, and over the nights to come – requiring sacrifice, trust and, very often, a big push out of their usual prayer comfort zone.

The prayer group that met on the evening I was airlifted to Perth, who later shared about the tangible presence of a spiritual battle that filled the room as they "pushed back against death" in prayer.

The mother of a friend, who was woken from the depth of sleep night after night during that week, prompted to get down on her knees by her bedside and pray passionately for the life of someone she'd never met.

The friend who vowed in faith and trust to fast of all food in prayer and petition while my condition remained unchanged on the ECMO life support.

The former work colleague who found it difficult to sleep, as the fear that I wasn't going to survive the night took hold. When she did finally succumb to sleep, after hours of faithful prayer, she was woken in the darkness of night by the audible beeping sound of hospital machinery filling her room. This friend – who has worked in a hospital setting for many years, and associates that beeping noise with life remaining in a patient – was at first frightened by the sound audibly filling her bedroom, but then exhilarated, as she understood God's reassurance that I was still alive.

The friend who'd been asking of God to embolden her in prayer publicly, who was now prompted to call the hospital in Perth and pray for me over the speaker phone, with two ICU nurses present as I lay in the coma.

These powerful interactions with the Living God are but a small number of the many stories shared with us of people being challenged in the way they prayed and the intensity of their prayer. When these faithful prayer warriors – both mature and new in their prayer lives – opened themselves in obedience to the prompting of God, He used them in His mighty and healing works. And in return, each of these people were encouraged, uplifted and exhilarated in spirit by the unique and powerful ways God convicted and spoke to them so personally.

Chapter Five

Jill's journal – Sunday 3rd April, early morning
You've survived the trauma of your first night of being critically ill on life support. As you were put into the induced coma, a groundswell of prayers began, with many people praying through the night for you. Our phones have started to ring and ping with texts constantly, letting us know that more and more people around Australia and overseas are praying for you, for your heart, and for the medical team treating you.

"It's early morning, and we're waiting for the sun to come up while you remain on ECMO". These words were handwritten by a nurse during my time in the coma, as part of an entry into a daily journal that was updated each shift by the many rotating nurses. Managing a critically ill patient on ECMO life support is incredibly labour intensive, with highly specialised medical staff required to provide around-the-clock care. In most cases, two ECMO-trained nurses will be in the room together at all times, responsible for monitoring the patient as well as the heart and lung machine and other life support measures (in my case a ventilator and an endotracheal breathing tube).

These nurses, on a rotating roster of twelve-hour shifts, became a lifeline for Matt and my parents – keeping them constantly updated over the phone on my condition and explaining the complexities of the machines, drips and monitoring processes. Crucially, they also provided a link between me in the coma and my family 150 kilometres away – although it seemed a desperately poor alternative to having my loved ones by my side in person, the skill, understanding and compassion of the ECMO nurses was deeply felt by Matt and my parents during that traumatic time of separation.

Matt's journal – Sunday 3rd April, morning
I'm very emotional and exhausted. I feel like I'm in a complete fog, and I can't understand what's happening. I just can't believe that you're on life support. I'm concerned for the wellbeing of your dad and mum, who are very upset and emotional too. Like me, they just desperately want you home healthy and fully recovered. They love you so very deeply. They've also been inundated with calls and messages of prayer and support. I'm keeping in constant contact with your parents, phoning them every time I talk to a nurse or doctor to give them an update. They comfort me a lot on the phone. But it's so hard to go through all of this and not even be able to hug them because of my isolation.

I still often feel an intense ache in my chest when I think of my family back at home in those hours and days of me being on life support. For a long time afterwards, there was a strange guilt that accompanied that ache – yes, I'd been critically ill in an induced coma, but I was also completely oblivious to, and unaffected by, the suffering that my loved ones were going through during that week. As someone who is normally very emotionally empathetic to the feelings and hurts of others, this was very hard for me to reconcile.

On the Sunday, day two of the coma, a close friend had delivered to our home a large rock which he placed in our back garden. It was positioned so Matt could see it through the window of our kitchen, where he now stood, the glass firmly closed to provide a quarantine barrier between him and our friend. On the rock our dear friend had written with bold, black marker the words *ON CHRIST THE SOLID ROCK I STAND*. Looking out of the window at that rock each day was a constant and necessary reminder to Matt that he wasn't relying on his own strength during this time – if he had, he would have well and truly fallen apart by now. Instead, he stood firmly in the strength of Christ, and His promise of a solid, unshakeable foundation.

The Lord is my rock, my fortress and my deliverer. My God is my rock, in whom I take refuge. He is my shield and the horn of my salvation, my stronghold. (Psalm 18:2)

That rock still stands in our garden today, an ongoing testament to the faithfulness of our Living Rock, Jesus, and to the strength-giving necessity of prayerful friends.

Matt's journal – Sunday 3rd April, afternoon

I've been blown away to find out how many churches and people are praying for you and our family – across WA and Australia, and even churches overseas. It is truly humbling. I've received so many messages and calls of love, support and prayers – you literally have armies of people praying you through this. It shows how many lives you've touched, and just how much you mean to so many people.

The tears of thankfulness I cried when I later learned of these heartful prayers were often and many. During the four years before 2022 I'd worked at a Christian school in Bunbury, serving in education assistance and literacy support in both the classroom and the library. Being involved with students from kindergarten through to Year 12, particularly in what I saw as the pastoral space of the library, had allowed me to connect with hundreds of students – and often their families – over the years. And now so many of these children, who'd become very dear to me, would pray for me at home, at the dinner table, and in their classes at school over the coming week. One teacher later described to me her amazement and emotion at hearing the boldness and passion of the prayers coming from the mouths and hearts of her year six students. It brought her to tears at the time, and did so for a long time afterwards. Many months after I woke from the coma, another staff member shared with Matt how her year two physical education class – children just six and seven years old – had spent a part of their sports lesson that week sitting in a group on the grass, taking turns one by one to pray for God's healing and protection over me. I can easily come to tears at the best of times, but the emotion that flooded me all those months later when I heard about the earnest and loving prayers of these precious children was pure and overwhelming.

Jesus said, "Let the little children come to me" (Matthew 19: 14)

Matt's journal – Sunday 3rd April, evening
Jesaia and Coby are coping well. I've explained things very simply to them, without all of the details, and they understand that you're in good care. They miss you though and ask if you'll be coming home tomorrow. I've cried a few times in front of

them, but mostly keep myself composed and strong for them. They need me.

"How did your boys deal with what was happening?" It's a question that was asked so often of me in the months after my being in the coma. I sometimes still get asked it now. Faith, family and friendship – an alliteration of the three major reasons our boys were supported so wholly during that time. While Matt would explain to them that their mum was sleeping deeply while a machine took over the work of her diseased heart, letting it rest, he never let on to our boys the life-threatening risks involved, the life-or-death situation of my illness. If Matt himself and my parents, in their wisdom and emotional maturity as adults, were struggling to comprehend that I might not survive the life-support, how could two young boys be burdened by the possibility of not seeing their mother again – without even being able to say goodbye? Even now, my heart still aches to write that sentence. Being able to actively take part in my boys' lives is one of the most emotional reasons I will never take my survival for granted. I'm in awe and gratitude of the fatherly strength it took Matt to protect our boys as he did of the dire reality of the situation – a strength which he received from his own, heavenly, Father. And although no parent would ever want their children to go through an experience like that, I praise God for the many ways in which our boys witnessed firsthand the practical expression of people living out their faith in love. Through the meals that poured in night after night, left quietly and lovingly on the doorstep of our home, accompanied by heartfelt notes. Through the gifts of toys, books and games that were bought and delivered to Jesaia and Coby, in a bid to take their minds off the situation and bring a smile to their young faces. Through the calls, messages, cards and letters, each containing compassionate words of encouragement and support. Through the chain of faithful, consistent prayer that strengthened and carried a family through the trauma, uncertainty and isolation of that week, and pushed back against dire medical odds.

My prayer remains… that our boys' experience of our mighty, living God – who loves, protects, heals and emboldens all of His children to come to Him personally in prayer – will fill them with confidence of truth, and strengthen and bring intimacy to their relationship with their Creator and Saviour.

Dad's text message to my phone – Sunday 3rd April, night
Hello precious Ab, fight on strongly our beautiful girl, you will win! We wish we could see you, and take your place. We love you SO incredibly much. Love Dad and Mum xoxo

Chapter Six

Jill's journal – Monday 4th April, morning
You are stable this morning on the life support, but very, very sick. Your heart is very weak, unable to keep your organs functioning without the help of the ECMO machine which is keeping you alive. Matt, your father and I are completely exhausted in mind, body and soul, but we praise and thank God that you have survived another night.

Matt's journal – Monday 4th April, morning
This morning I got to have two video calls to your mobile phone. One of the ICU nurses in your isolation pod used the calls to show me you and your bed, as well as all of the equipment and tubes around you keeping you alive. It was very overwhelming at first, and I cried when I saw you like that. As hard as it was, I was very relieved to finally be able to see you, to connect with you, even in such an inadequate way. You looked peaceful, and your face was beauty to me.
You are being very well looked after. You always have two nurses in the room with you, so you're never alone. It gives me so much comfort knowing our Lord is right there in the room

with you, never leaving you. Especially given how hard it is for me not being there by your side.

A few days after waking from the coma, a dear friend sent a video through to my phone in ICU – a montage of people from our church, waving, smiling (underneath their masks – eye smiles, my nurse and I called them) and sending their messages of love. It was so precious and filled my weak but healing body with gladness. A short time after coming home from hospital, I was searching for the video in my phone's gallery and came across a number of photos taken of me on life support, which had been sent to Matt on that first Monday. An unexpected shock ripped through me, my heart hammering and hands shaking as I stared at an image of myself in the coma. It was both visually and emotionally confronting, especially as I thought of Matt receiving these pictures of his wife at that time, unable to be by my side. And yet... as I looked closely at all of the medical machinery surrounding me, the tubes, the hospital gown, the swollen face and limbs, a body wracked with illness, I could see clearly what Matt had written in his journal that Monday. Despite the medical chaos wreaking havoc inside my body, *I looked completely at peace.* Deep in the darkness of the coma, I was resting in the arms of the One who gave me life. As confronting as that photo was, it remained a powerful image of a daughter of God, lying in human frailty, in His complete and tender protection, care and peace.

I will lie down and sleep in peace, for you alone, O Lord, make me dwell in safety. (Psalm 4:8)

Matt's journal – Monday 4th April, afternoon

After lunch, Jordan and Jen [brother and sister-in-law] came to pick up Jesaia to walk with him to the park for a kick of the footy, as it's his first day out of isolation. I cried while talking to them about how much I missed you, which set off their crying too (all through the front door – me standing inside, both of them outside). Later, your Aunty Jacqui called me to suggest that I could ask the nurses to play some worship music to you while you're in the coma. So I found a few lovely instrumental worship playlists on YouTube, because I know how calming you find it listening to this music at home. I wonder if you can hear it? In the depth of your coma, does your spirit rejoice in hearing it?

As it turns out, I did hear it. What a gift that music would prove to be, bringing calm and peace to my darkest days ahead…

Jill's journal – Monday 4th April, afternoon
Matt is still unwell with covid. His throat became even worse overnight, red, painful, with swollen glands. Your father and I do all we can to support him and the boys, all at a safe distance. We phone each other frequently. We wait helplessly and pray.

That was another layer of the many challenges Matt was facing during that week – he himself was unwell with covid, exacerbated without doubt by the extreme stress and emotion of the circumstances, and a lack of sleep or even rest. Every part of his body was under assault – physically, emotionally and mentally. And yet… in his complete weakness and lack of control, Matt's total reliance on God's strength and provision was profound, in a way that he'd never experienced before.

Many months later, as a sense of normalcy in everyday activity started to slowly return to our family, Matt would share that he actually missed that place of complete vulnerability and intimacy with God that he'd come to at that time, during a week where he was repeatedly – both literally and spiritually – brought to his knees in total submission and surrender to the only One in control of both the present and the future.

Chapter Seven

Jill's journal – Tuesday 5th April, afternoon
I went to work today – I needed routine to keep my mind and emotions together. While driving to work, waiting at the traffic lights and praying, I was given a very clear 'picture' of a big Jesus holding a little Abbey in His strong arms. In the image, you could physically feel His skin, and the warmth and strength of His arms.

What an incredible gift my mum received that morning, as she cried out to God for reassurance, comfort and strength to get through another challenging day of the unknown. It profoundly impacted her in that moment, and in the days to come – a tangible reassurance that her child was being held, protected and carried by our Heavenly Father. As Matt would later describe it, God wasn't watching the situation from a distance. He wasn't even just sitting in the corner of my ICU room. Instead He rolled up His sleeves, scooped me into His strong arms, and carried me through it! Despite my closest loved ones not being allowed by my side as I lay in the coma, I was *never* alone.

Months later, my mum called me, excited and overwhelmed after coming across an artwork titled 'Jesus Saves' by UK artist Debbie Clark that almost exactly reflected the picture she'd seen that morning in April at the traffic lights – strong, calm, compassionate Jesus holding a young girl (who looked very much like I did as a dark-haired, hazel-eyed child) in His loving, secure arms. It still brings me to tears of awe to know that, amongst the beeps and life-support machinery of a hospital room, that girl was me.

I have made you and I will carry you (Isaiah 46:4)

Matt's journal – Tuesday 5th April, afternoon

You've remained in a stable condition this morning. Your circulation, skin colour and temperature are all good. The specialists and doctors did an echo ultrasound to test if your heart has regained any strength. They found you've made a very small improvement compared to when you went onto the ECMO machine, so they're able to slightly reduce the level of life support. We're all greatly encouraged by the small improvement, because for the first time you're going in the right direction. I feel more peaceful today that you'll make a full recovery.

And then…

Jill's journal – Tuesday 5th April, evening
This evening, one of the doctors has given Matt a brutal report on your health – you're the sickest patient in ICU, your heart is completely diseased and not improving at the rate it needs to, you might be on life support for weeks, and your other organs are at risk of deteriorating. We've gone from elation that you've shown a slight improvement, to devastation at the doctor's report.

Matt would later share that, during that time, when each phone call would seem to bring more news he struggled to comprehend, he would repeat out loud, over and over "God is mighty to save". What a humble, incredibly faithful declaration of trust. Trust in uncertainty. Trust in humility through a complete lack of control. Trust that our God is indeed mighty to save, when the dark thoughts of a future without his wife tempted Matt to consider otherwise.

Dad's text message to my phone – Tuesday 5th April, night
Sleep peacefully tonight my love. You are a gorgeous girl. All our love, Dad and Mum xoxo

Chapter Eight

Matt's journal – Wednesday 6th April, morning

You're now going into your fourth day on life support. I've had a call from the cardiologist at the hospital, Dr James Lambert, letting me know your doctors will be performing a heart biopsy on you this afternoon around 3pm. They'll be taking a sample of heart tissue to test for a particular type of inflammation that would need a change in treatment. Dr Lambert explained that, because your condition is very fragile, there are a number of risks in performing the biopsy. The main risk is causing a hole in your heart, but there's also the risk of moving you with all of the life support equipment from ICU to theatre and back again. Your parents let Jamie [their church pastor] know, and I let Richard [our pastor] know, so they can spread the word and ask people to pray specifically for this biopsy.

It was such a difficult phone call, as Dr Lambert said you're still in a critical condition and your heart is still very diseased, but if you stay on the ECMO machine beyond one to two weeks other serious problems will begin to accumulate. You've already gained around 10kg of fluid buildup, which they're removing from your body. Dr Lambert was clear that they're preparing for all scenarios when it comes to weaning you off the life support, with one scenario being that your heart still won't be strong enough to support you. He actually told me that you're the sickest ICU patient in hospital at the moment. I feel scared again after that phone call, and suddenly the relief and optimism we all felt from yesterday's small improvement is under threat.

The sickest ICU patient in hospital. Considering that intensive care units are literally filled with people in critical and life-threatening conditions, that unwanted title was incredibly hard to comprehend, both by Matt when he heard the words at the time, and for me when I was told some time after the coma. Many months later, a friend would tell us that she'd sat watching the TV news one evening while I was on life support, reading from the screen the daily statistics of patients in ICU in WA with covid (there were eight at the time), thinking "I can't believe I *know* one of those people". It was incredibly surreal, she admitted. We just don't expect to be connected so intimately with the news stories we often only half-listen to as we prepare dinner and wind down from the day. Now, though, I was one of those numbers on the screen, and I was the sickest of the sick. It would be one of many statistics bound closely to my illness and recovery… and yet God – the Master Physician - doesn't work in the business of statistics, no matter how confronting they are.

Jill's journal – Wednesday 6th April, afternoon
Before your biopsy, the cardiologist told Matt that your heart is so completely diseased and inflamed that wherever he takes the sample from will show him what he needs to see. It was a virtual 'military operation' to get you and your life-saving machinery successfully downstairs to the operating theatre. Now we all hold our breath and pray!

It's actually been my worst day during this time, and I was a mess by lunchtime. And then I had three visitors – all at the same time, all bearing meals – to bless me with their support. All three prayed with me for your biopsy, and for the doctors who are doing the operation.

These three women – who knew my mum but weren't familiar with each other – were all open and obedient to God's prompting on that day to stop whatever they were doing and drive to my parents' house at the same time on my mum's self-described 'worst day'. It was after lunch and my dad wasn't at home, having driven to a local oval with Jesaia and Coby to kick the footy. Both boys were now fully recovered from their covid, free from their required isolation and desperate for some space and fresh air in which to run and distract their minds. Mum had stayed at home, struggling with the emotional enormity of the situation, when she collapsed onto the floor in floods of heaving tears. She hadn't contacted any of the women but, with God's leading, all three knew at the same moment that my mum needed their tangible support and prayer. One of the women – my aunty – would later admit that, after arriving at my parents' home, she actually thought I must have died, such was the emotional state my mum was found in. At the exact same time that I, along with all of my life-support machinery, was being carefully transferred through the hospital and down into the operating theatre for surgery, these three beautiful ladies – meeting each other for the first time - prayed with my mum, bringing her the comfort, strength and peace she so desperately needed in that moment.

That day, that moment, was yet another example of God's people being attuned to His prompting, and showing obedience and trust in acting out His direction. My mum will never forget that day – and, through the spiritual encouragement of hearing this story, neither will I.

Matt's journal – Wednesday 6th April, evening
While you were having your biopsy, I listened to worship music and prayed. Late in the afternoon, the hospital phoned to say you were now back in your ICU room, the procedure to take a biopsy had gone well, and you had remained stable right throughout. Praise God! Another moment of relief.

It's funny the little things that can often stand out in our minds and hearts as being so important to us. That Wednesday was the day a beautiful friend of ours took the time to collect a pair of new football boots that had been waiting for collection at our local sports store – ordered online by me a number of weeks before – and drop them off at the front door of our home for our oldest boy Jesaia. The start of footy season was rapidly approaching, and those boots provided our son with a much-needed reassurance of normality.

Love and kindness can so often be found in the smallest of details.

Matt's journal – Wednesday 6th April, night
I've been regularly checking in with Jesaia and Coby to see how they're feeling, and to give them lots of hugs. They both miss you very much. After dinner we watched a movie together (Paddington 2, which we know you always enjoy) because I just really felt like snuggling down with them on the couch.

Love and comfort can so often be found in the simplest of moments.

Chapter Nine

Matt's journal – Thursday 7th April, morning
I had a much better sleep last night and feel the best I've felt since becoming unwell with covid a week ago. My body still feels very tired, but my cough has improved. I'm so desperate to be completely well again, so there's nothing stopping me from being with you in the hospital as soon as possible.
There's no news yet about the biopsy results, but the ICU nurses said you had another stable night and your vital signs are good, which was a relief to hear after your procedure yesterday. They also told me the doctors are going to perform another weaning test, where they reduce the level of life support and monitor your heart using ultrasound to see how it responds. This will happen this afternoon around 3pm and will take a couple of hours. I straight away told Richard (our pastor), and your dad let Jamie (their pastor) know, so the prayer troops can be rallied again to pray specifically for this test.
After the phone conversation yesterday with the cardiologist Dr Lambert I feel a sense of urgency that this test today needs to show a significant improvement in your heart's recovery and strength. You've been on ECMO for five days now. If this test

finds no improvement, or only a small one, the situation will seem very dire.

So now it's another nervous wait – waiting for the test to be performed, waiting for a doctor to call me with the results – and urgently praying for you to have made a significant improvement.

Jill's journal – Thursday 7th April, afternoon
People around the world are on their knees praying for your condition. It's become a true prayer 'movement' that has grown daily.

And then...

Matt's journal – Thursday 7th April, evening
An incredible answer to prayer! The test has found your heart has recovered to about 50 percent strength and is therefore strong enough for you to be taken off the ECMO machine tomorrow, as long as you have a stable night tonight! I received the news over the phone from Dr Chris Allen, an ICU Intensivist and ECMO specialist, who's part of the team looking after you. Dr Allen told me you'll still remain in the induced coma on the breathing machine for up to a week, until it's also safe to wean you off that as well. Based on the test results, Dr Allen said he's optimistic for your recovery and, while you

aren't out of the woods by any means, this is your first big step towards that.
This is such good news! After all of the bad news over the past week it's almost a shock, and is taking a while to sink in. Praise God for the fruit of so many people continually praying for you and your full recovery!

Your full recovery. Three powerful words that point to the faithfulness and boldness of people's prayer during that time. Despite the critical situation, the risks and potential side effects, so many people prayed confidently and boldly that I wouldn't 'just survive', but that I would be completely restored, physically and medically – my heart fully healed, my internal organs spared of long-term damage, my limbs intact. In the face of an often bleak outlook, these prayers petitioned for nothing less than my full recovery, and I'll forever be humbled and overwhelmed with gratitude by that.

Jill's journal – Thursday 7th April, evening
There is so much joy as the stunning news gets out on all the many prayer lines and groups! Praise God over and over!! Two people contacted me independently of each other this evening to share that they were given a 'picture' while praying of a mountain which must be brought down – the mountain of virus

attacking your heart. This brings much encouragement following the test results, and gives us a focus on which to pray.

Dad's text message to my phone – Thursday 7th April, night
You're winning the battle, our beautiful Ab! You're a treasure, we love you and praise God so much for you! Hundreds and hundreds of people are upholding you in prayer – they all love you like we do! See you soon, our precious luv. Love you heaps, Dad and Mum xoxo

Chapter Ten

Friday 8th April. The date that Matt would later describe as "the day God's miracles and answers to prayers started flying in!" This was the day I'd be brought off the ECMO machine, the intensive life support which had been functioning as my heart for the past six days. The understanding was that I'd still remain in the coma, on a ventilator, for days to come, but it would be a massive step forward to release me from this life support of last resort.

Except that God was powerfully bringing down those mountains, one after the other, and He wasn't going to stop at just the ECMO machine...

Matt's journal – Friday 8th April, morning

Today is my final day of isolation, and I'm feeling much better. It's also exactly one week since I last saw you.

When I phoned the hospital earlier this morning to find out how you went overnight, I found out the doctors had just seen you and are preparing to take you off the ECMO machine sooner rather than later. It was originally planned to happen this afternoon, but you've developed a small bleed where the tubes went into your leg, and so they've brought it forward.

Not long after, a doctor phoned me to explain the surgery and ask for my consent. Removing you from the ECMO machine will involve making an incision in the groin area to repair the vein and two arteries that are connected to the tubes that have been drawing and returning your blood from and to your body. Again, we wait and pray.

And this is where I re-enter the story.

That's always been a deeply strange and unsettling thought, given I've been at the centre of the past week's events. But I've been unaware, oblivious, immersed in a coma while the days moved on. It's been a week filled with panic, confusion, uncertainty, disbelief and tears for my loved ones – but also prayer, strength, encouragement and hope. For me though, it's been void of anything – no memories, trauma or even tangible darkness. Like falling asleep and waking up the next morning – or in this case, the next Friday. Just a blip in time. Until now.

Because now, on this seventh day, I can see things. Images that will return in my memory as time goes on. It starts with the faces. The smiling, laughing faces of children, playing in a village which, on later reflection, seems to be located somewhere in Africa. The beautiful dark-skinned faces of women – who might be the children's mothers – that slowly turn into the faces of lions, in a dizzying circular motion of colour. More animals, in the form of tigers – in this vision, young boys of Asian heritage run away from the tigers, always one step ahead, still laughing. Another image, another group of boys running, this time away from a number of men who are chasing them down an alleyway. There's no laughter this time. The men leap on the boys, who manage to escape after a quick struggle. This vision is the only one that I find dangerous and distressing in the moment – wanting it to stop, but powerless to do so. Other visions are more peaceful, including the one of the elderly, weathered man sitting on the verandah of what appears to be a traditional Australian homestead, the house surrounded by gum trees and gardens. In between the images are visions of more gardens – mostly roses, with row after row of flowers – as well as fireworks, both of which explode with colour. The multicolours dissolve one image into the next, in a kaleidoscopic spin that will later plague my nighttime when I'm awake from the coma. The final vision I recall is again filled with smiling faces – those of young women with teased peroxide blonde hair and heavy makeup, laughing as they call out "Here we go again". And then the cycle of images starts again, and I feel strangely accepting of the fact that, although I want to leave this confusing world of interchanging faces, animals, flowers and colours, it isn't time just yet.

Many months later, I would tell the ECMO specialist of the images I saw. While it's impossible to say exactly when I would have experienced them, the fact I could remember them so vividly after being brought out of the coma indicates they likely happened on that Friday, the day of returning to consciousness. I've often wondered if the words "Here we go again" that I remembered from one of the visions was in fact spoken in my ICU room, as the medical staff slowly brought me out of the coma in stages that day. The images feel like a bridge between a week of darkness and oblivion, and my awareness of joining the living world again.

Matt's journal – Friday 8th April, late morning

You're free from the ECMO machine!! I've just had a phone call from Dr Lambert the cardiologist, who said you're now back in your ICU room, and your heart is coping well with being off the ECMO machine and doing all the blood pumping itself. His words were "Abbey flew off the ECMO machine!" Praise God! The surgery to patch your arteries went well, with Dr Lambert commenting that your arteries were better than most people's! It's such an answer to prayer, and a huge step forward in your recovery. After your condition and the whole situation seemed so dire less than 48 hours ago, your heart is now strong enough to support you, and you're off the ECMO machine!

Two hours later...

Matt's journal – Friday 8th April, afternoon
I've been prepared that you might still have to remain on the breathing machine and in the induced coma for up to a week after coming off ECMO. But now, only a couple of hours after being taken off the life-support machine, an ICU nurse has just called me to say they might try to wake you up this afternoon, to see if you can tolerate coming off the breathing machine! They can't guarantee it will happen today, but they're going to monitor you to decide if you're ready.

Jill's journal – Friday 8th April, afternoon
We're now seeing those 'mountains' we've been praying against crumbling everywhere! The mountain of coming off ECMO, the mountain of bringing you out of the coma – they're all coming down! The specialists are amazed at this dramatic turnaround in your condition. Your heart is now functioning well and Dr Chris Allen has told Matt several times that this is extraordinary, considering how very sick you were just a day or two ago. It's obvious we have witnessed a miracle! All glory and praise to our mighty God!!

And then the journal entry that, to this day, still brings me to tears to read. The raw relief and almost disbelief felt by Matt to finally hear the voice of his wife – weak, terribly disoriented, but awake. Alive.

Matt's journal – Friday 8th April, late afternoon
I was quietly folding washing in our bedroom listening to the song 'Way Maker' when my phone rang, and to my huge surprise it was your number! The ICU nurse Susan had used your mobile to call me to say they'd brought you out of the coma! I couldn't believe you were actually awake! The nurse told me you were agitated, disorientated from waking up in a strange room, and hallucinating from the heavy medications you've been on. She assured me this was a very normal response when coming out of a coma, and asked if I could talk to you to help comfort you and calm you down. Your words were slurred and difficult to understand, but I was just ecstatic to hear your voice and know that you were awake! You seemed to be upset by all the tubes and equipment in the room, and something about the ceiling was bothering you. I tried to comfort you as best I could, and told you that I loved you, which you were able to say back to me! After a few minutes the nurse ended the phone call, and I collapsed onto the floor sobbing and giving thanks to God. I cannot explain the relief I felt to know you are awake and now completely off life support.

I immediately phoned your parents to let them know the incredible news, and they were ecstatic too! Then I sent some messages out to people letting them know you're awake, and I started receiving so many texts and calls as the news began to spread. Everyone is so thrilled and relieved, and giving thanks and praise to God!

"I love you too". Four incredibly precious words that Matt, in his deepest moments of fear and darkness, thought he might never hear from his wife again. But now he was on the floor of our bedroom, sobbing and praising God after I spoke those words to him during our first phone conversation after waking from the coma. An exchange of love which I have no memory of, due to a mind distressed by medication and post-coma trauma. But God shows His grace and mercy to us in so many ways, including through the gentle words of a husband, and the lyrics of a worship song proclaiming His promises. In that moment, His spirit settled my turmoiled soul.

Matt's text message to family and friends - Friday 8th April, 5pm

My wife is awake!!!!!!!! The Lord has delivered Abbey and His faithful, strong arms have carried her through!!!! I got to speak with her to help calm her down as she woke from the coma because she was very confused and disoriented. I am speechless and so grateful to God!!

Chapter Eleven

I've often said that on that Friday – the end of my week on life support, when so many were celebrating and praising God for my healing – what felt like a living nightmare was just beginning for me. The feeling of sickness and pain ripping through every part of my body when I first opened my eyes was all-consuming in its ferocity. From the severe aching to the intense nausea and dizziness, there wasn't a single part of me that didn't feel under attack. I had a cannula attached to each wrist, and when I tried to lift my head to look around the room, the many tubes and wires leading into my neck, chest and groin restricted my movement and created the claustrophobic sensation of being pinned to the bed. Severely impacted by the medications that had kept me in the coma, nothing seemed upright or stable – the room appeared tilted, objects were in a constant state of motion, my bed rolled as if on wheels. "Help me, somebody help me", I moaned over and over again, the sounds difficult to form, my words slurred. My body felt so ravaged by sickness, pain and weakness that I truly thought I must be dying. Of course I had no understanding how close I'd, in actual fact, come to death over the past week, and that, despite how wretched I was feeling now, I was already significantly improved from my most critical point. Because absolutely nothing made sense. The room was unfamiliar, the bed definitely wasn't my own from home, the sound of persistent beeping filled my ears and – most confusingly of all – I recognised no one. So much research into comas confirms the value of loved ones being able to sit by the patient's bedside, talking to them and giving physical touch. That human presence of a loved one is also incredibly important to the patient's state of mind when they're brought out of a coma, providing much-needed familiarity and reassurance. My brain was already deeply confused – I had no understanding of why I was there, or even where 'there' was, and no memory of how I'd gotten to this place. The only other living creature in my room was covered head to toe in PPE, preventing my addled mind from comprehending this nurse as human. I desperately needed a familiar face to offer context to my situation, to hear the comforting words of someone who knew me and loved me. The hand of my husband, son or parent to hold mine. Without that, it was a situation of utter confusion mixed with critical illness. And that's when I started to panic.

IN THE MORNING CAME THE LIGHT

It was the music that finally calmed me. "Try putting on some worship songs", Matt had suggested to my nurse on the phone, and now, as she sat in the corner of the room, searching for a playlist on her computer, music began filtering into my conscience, encouraging my memory to again latch onto something familiar. "Way maker... miracle worker... promise keeper... light in the darkness... my God... that is who you are". I knew that tune - from just recently! - from the swirling images, and the kaleidoscopic colours, and the urge to be freed of the repeated cycle of laughing people, running feet and wild animal faces. Without even knowing it, the words had provided peace in the darkness of the coma, and now they again brought me much-needed comfort. "Light in the darkness"... I was going to have to call on that Light – at times plead with that Light – over and over throughout the coming days.

That powerful song 'Way Maker', written by Nigerian gospel singer Sinach, will forever be incredibly special to my husband and me. The lyrics provided my first flash of memory – which I'm certain came from hearing that song of promise while in the coma – and brought me a supernatural peace in that initial moment of intense panic. Later, I would find out that a family very dear to ours, who'd moved interstate a few months before I became sick, would sing 'Way Maker' together every night that I was in the coma, as a declaration of trust in who our Almighty God is. Miracle worker. Promise keeper. The Light in the darkness. Each member of the family of six would choose one person to pray for – myself, Matt, Jesaia, Coby, my dad Struan, or my mum Jill – and commit us to God as they praised him through song. To this day, every time I listen to 'Way Maker' (as I especially love to do when I'm out walking in His creation most mornings) I think of this precious family, and the way so many just like them prayed my family and me through that week, and into that first horrendous night.

As time marches on, the practical details of that first horrendous night out of the coma start to fade, although the intense feelings of distress, confusion and loneliness never do. The overriding memory of that middle-of-the-night darkness is the sickening sensation of my hospital bed rolling backwards down a hill in a never-ending motion, my body pinned down and unable to get off.

"Lord, please make this stop! I beg you!"

"My God, you have the power to make this stop! Please, I beg you!"

"Lord, I can't bear this anymore! Please, please, please God. Make it stop, I beg you!"

I'm still not sure whether I cried these pleas out loud, or whether they were screamed inside my head – either way, I begged God in my ICU room that night to release me from the nauseating dizziness of feeling like I was upside down in constant motion. And yet... it didn't stop. There wasn't immediate relief, I didn't suddenly sink into much-needed sleep that would blot out the pain and sickness. It continued, but my God – who is always listening – gave me the strength to keep on crying out to him in my weakness.

Months later, I would be reading my bible and come across the words of the apostle Paul, a follower of Jesus who was no stranger to pain and affliction:

Three times I pleaded with the Lord to take it away from me. But He said to me, "My grace is sufficient for you, for my power is made perfect in weakness." (2 Corinthians 12:8)

My hands began to shake and I started crying tears of understanding as I read the passage. It was as though Paul himself had been an observer in my room that dark night, his words perfectly capturing the necessity and power of surrender in the anguish of the moment. For in that moment – confused and disoriented, lying attached by tubes to a hospital bed in an ICU room, tormented by an all-consuming sickness that wouldn't be relieved and a constant rolling motion that wouldn't stop – I was well and truly at my weakest and most vulnerable. I felt I had nothing left in me. And yet when I couldn't plead anymore, little did I know that so many others that night were interceding in prayer for me. And the power of Christ – made perfect in my weakness – rested on me.

Chapter Twelve

Jill's journal – Saturday 9th April, afternoon
You've spoken to Matt and us several times on the phone today, and it was so wonderful to hear your voice! You did sound strained and not yourself, although you're on many medications and steroids so this is very understandable. You don't understand where you are or why Matt isn't with you, and you just want to leave and come home. When we tell you that people from around the world have been praying for you, you blankly ask why they would do that, and we realise you have no memory of what's happened to you over the past 10 days. We have to be careful with how much we tell you, as we understand that none of this makes sense to you and could distress you. We're concerned now for your state of mind, and your agitation at what's happening. But we continue to praise God for your incredible physical improvement, and that your heart continues to pump faithfully. And even though you don't yet understand, we tell you again that we have witnessed a miracle!

Matt's journal – Saturday 9th April, evening
I'm still testing positive to covid, which I'm really disappointed about because I so desperately want to visit you. You spoke to

me on the phone at about 1am overnight and then again at 7am this morning. You hadn't been able to sleep, and you were feeling very anxious and agitated to get off your bed and out of your ICU room. We had a long video call on your phone in the late morning, and it was incredible to see you free of the life support equipment and all of the breathing tubes, although you still have cannulas in your neck and arms.

It felt amazing to me to be talking with you after all you'd been through over the past nine days since I'd dropped you off at Bunbury Hospital! I told you that you were doing so well, and that I'm very proud of you. You got to see Jesaia and Coby for the first time during this call too, which was very emotional. Your voice sounded robotic though, and you were still clearly unaware of how sick you've been.

You needed lots of time talking on the phone over video calls throughout the afternoon and evening to help comfort you, as you're still feeling very anxious and disoriented. Dr Allen explained to me that the way you're feeling is normal, and is caused by the withdrawal effects of coming off the medication that was keeping you asleep in the coma. During one of our calls, I suggested some worship songs that the nurse in your room could play to help calm you. We even sung a bit of the song "Oh Praise the Name" together over the phone.

Later on, you said that when you closed your eyes you could see colours and visions, which was distressing you. You've now been given medication to help calm and sedate you, in the hope that you'll get some sleep tonight.

Sleep, unfortunately, did not come to me on that Saturday night either. Instead, it was a night that I can only describe as one of intense spiritual darkness, a time that lay uneasily in my thoughts for a long time afterwards. As Matt had written in his journal, my mind was relentlessly tortured by visions and hallucinations – some of which were connected to those I'd seen in the coma, all of which made no sense whatsoever. The hospital room in which I'd laid for the past week was in what's called Pod Four, a corner area of the ICU that was now a strict isolation zone. (An interesting side note... a close friend had worked in PR years before, and had been responsible for promoting the newly built state-of-the-art isolation pods at Fiona Stanley Hospital to the media. Little did she know her friend would be lying in a coma in one of those very rooms some years later.) Each individual room was surrounded by walls made of glass that could frost for privacy, or defrost to be seen through, at the touch of a button by any one of my medical staff. Most of the time the glass was frosted, which made any movement outside the room appear distorted, even to the clearest of minds. My perception was far from coherent however, and the constant passing of medical staff in the corridor outside my room throughout that long Saturday night caused me huge distress. I heard the thudding sounds of running footsteps, and visions of young boys being chased in an alleyway – just as I'd seen in the coma – bombarded my mind. Over and over I pleaded with the nurse in my room to help them.

"Who are those people being chased out there? Why isn't anyone helping them? You need to help them!"

The nurse repeatedly reassured me that no one was in danger, that there weren't any boys being chased outside my room – but with no understanding of where "outside my room" even was, and the visions relentlessly filling my mind, I couldn't believe her.

Another torment that night were the psychedelic explosions of colour that filled my eyes every time I closed them – like inside one of those kaleidoscopes I'd played with as a child, but without the fun. It made sleep entirely impossible, and even resting my eyes shut caused a rush of colour and subsequent nausea. By this point, I'd not slept for thirty-six hours straight – an irony, I'd realise later, after having been 'asleep' for six days straight before that in the coma.

I was also intensely thirsty in a way that I'd never experienced before, with my mouth completely dried out, making it difficult to even form my words. To avoid liquid potentially entering my lungs I wasn't allowed to drink water, so I was given ice chips to suck on – the gloved nurse feeding them into my mouth on the end of a spoon. Each small mouthful of ice chips would give me a desperately sweet moment of hydrating relief before the thirst and dry mouth would immediately return, leaving me literally begging for more.

The glass wall between my isolation room and the next contained a sliding door, that could be opened to create one large space. As all medical staff in Pod Four were wearing head-to-toe PPE, my nurse and the nurse next door could, at times, slide open the door and move between the rooms, providing each other with support and much-needed company on what was an otherwise very isolating twelve-hour shift. Later, I would feel comfort and a sense of joy in listening to the two nurses chatter together about everyday topics, a taste of normality in a completely abnormal situation. But in the middle of this dark night, when the nurse from the room next to mine crossed over the threshold for a chat, every sound, every word, felt like a rocket exploding in my head, building in persistence and intensity until I couldn't take it anymore, begging the nurse to stop talking and restore quiet in my room.

When that door slid open and a press of the button defrosted the glass separating my ICU room from the next, I could see the patient lying in his own bed next door, staring intently at me. Unable to fully turn my body away because of the tubes, I would avert my eyes for a few moments before glancing back to find him still staring, expressionless and refusing to look away. I know full well now that this patient was very unwell himself, and obviously had no intimidating intent or even awareness of his actions at all. But in that moment, my confused mind was plagued with uncertainty, anxiety and heightened emotion, and I felt incredibly vulnerable and helpless. Never more did I crave my husband's comforting presence by my bedside than in that moment.

A relentless, uncontrollable cough also wracked my weakened body that night. It would take hold of me with a ferocious force, leaving me gasping for breath and causing my already aching head to throb with the intensity. It was impossible to contain and, even in my illness, I felt strangely and acutely self-conscious of my contagion. Despite my confused state, I did understand that I'd had – still had – covid, and that I wasn't allowed home, nor were my family allowed to visit me. So in my desperation, I decided that my cough was the key to showing my nurses that I was recovered enough to leave hospital, and if I could therefore just refrain from coughing, they'd let me go home and I could be with my family again. I would turn my head into my pillow, away from the direction of my nurse, frantically trying to stifle the next wracking cough that would inevitably take over my entire body. In my mind I'd imagine the nurse thinking, "What a shame, she just coughed again. She won't be able to go home after all". And another wave of feeling trapped, desperate and alone would crash over me.

Jill's journal – Saturday 9th April, middle of the night
Our precious Abbey... so many people are continuing to pray for your protection. God is surrounding you with His strength when you have none and are vulnerable.

"I wish he'd just left me to die."

Eight words that caused me a lot of guilt in the weeks after I uttered them. I'd cried this in the height of my anguish to the ICU Intensivist Dr Chris Allen, after he'd explained to me that my husband Matt's actions in getting me to hospital more than a week earlier had set in motion a course of action that would save my life. A feeling of shame washed over me later when I understood how faithfully so many people had committed to my recovery and survival during that week on life support – through skilled medical hands, through loving care and sacrifice, through so much prayer. For now though I couldn't comprehend that. In that moment, relief from the all-consuming pain and sickness in any way was my primal desire, whatever that looked like.

Even now, whenever I think back to that night, the feeling that still overwhelmingly stands out is that of loneliness – feeling achingly, completely isolated in my state of physical sickness and psychological torment. I had no one familiar in my room – and the nurse that was there appeared more alien than human in her PPE – I couldn't physically escape, and nothing was relieving my state. I felt so incredibly lonely and trapped.

And yet, I was never alone. That night, many faithful people continued to commit me in prayer to the God who promises He will always be with us (John 16:32). Despite the fact that I was now out of the 'danger zone' – off ECMO and the ventilator, and out of the coma – a friend was woken with a start at 3.30am on that Saturday night, prompted strongly to get out of bed and pray fervently for me, despite not knowing exactly why. After all, shouldn't he have been celebrating my incredible recovery from a near-fatal illness (which he was!), and now resting peacefully after many nights of broken sleep? And yet my friend was discerning to God's prompting of prayer, fully trusting and obedient to His direction in that moment. When I found out about this many months later, I shared with my friend that, despite not being able to recall many details of that first forty-eight hours post-coma, I vividly remembered the early-morning hour between 3am and 4am on that second night as being the darkest of the dark.

My nurse had gone on her meal break, meaning the nurse caring for the patient in the room next to mine was now responsible for us both during that hour. In my confused state I now felt incredibly vulnerable, repeatedly asking when my nurse would be returning. Appearing indifferent to my growing distress, the nurse from next door refused to give an answer, instead impatiently telling me that my carer would be back in my room "whenever she's ready". Given I was already so disoriented and completely powerless in my situation, the lack of compassion and understanding in his response added to my intense loneliness. I was also intensely thirsty, my mouth and throat completely parched of any moisture. In a state of desperation I begged for ice chips to momentarily relieve the thirst, but was told I couldn't have any until my nurse returned – whenever that would be – and could then monitor me. Fixated by the time, staring at the clock on the wall of my hospital room, I watched the minutes slide by slowly, painfully – weakened, vulnerable and crying out to God in pain, sickness, thirst and confusion. And He heard me and He cared for me. He cared for me through the discerning friend who committed the early hour of 3am that Sunday morning to pray for me, at the exact time I most needed it. He cared for me through the Christian nurse who'd unexpectedly took over the night shift when her colleague became unwell from the restrictive PPE. She also looked and sounded very much like a dear friend of mine, bringing me a craved-for sense of comfort and reassurance in her familiarity. And He cared for me in the words that continued to play in my mind throughout that night, remembered from the coma – clear with promise, despite the chaos and confusion of everything else…

Even when I don't see it, you're working
Even when I don't feel it, you're working
You never stop, you never stop working…
You are Way maker, miracle worker, promise keeper
Light in the darkness
My God, that is who You are ('Way Maker') [1]

Chapter Thirteen

And then in the morning – Sunday – came the light.

Physically, mentally and emotionally, it was as though a spiritual hold had been broken, and a battle had been won. Despite not having had even a minute's sleep again for the second night in a row, by the time my day nurse Georgia began her twelve-hour shift in my room at around 7am, I was experiencing a lightness I hadn't felt since waking from the coma. The veil that had cloaked me in darkness, fear and loneliness for the past forty-eight hours had lifted, and I now rested in complete peace. It felt incredible.

One of the first - and most profound, given the state I'd been in – actions my nurse Georgia took that early Sunday morning was to take a black marker and handwrite her name in large capital letters across the front of her blue PPE gown. The impact of such a seemingly simple action was huge. Until now, it had been impossible to identify or remember the names of the nurses who had revolved through my isolation room in twelve-hour shifts. Not only had my mind been incapable of such understanding, the full-body PPE – caps covering the hair, eye goggles, clear plastic face shields, surgical masks, gowns, gloves and enclosed shoes – wreaked havoc with my recognition of the medical staff who were caring for me. The ICU Intensivist Dr Allen, who would visit me in my room daily, wore a bright orange surgical mask, which differentiated him from the other doctors and nurses wearing white facial coverings. The mask had the appearance of a duck's beak, and for the first two days after the coma, in my state of confusion and delirium, I actually thought a walking, talking duck was standing by my bedside each day. So now, when nurse Georgia wrote her name across the front of her blue gown, a desperately needed human connection with my carer began.

The second simple act Georgia did was open the blinds in my room, filling it with light and enabling me to take in properly for the first time my surroundings. It's very possible the window coverings had been opened at other times and I was too unwell to register, but for now, I felt a literal and metaphorical light envelop my space, and in a small way I started to finally make sense of where I was.

I remember Georgia also turned on the TV in my ICU room for the first time as I attempted to eat a small amount of breakfast, filling my room with the sounds of *Weekend Sunrise*. The impact of the sheer normality of hearing chattering and laughter from the hosts interacting with each other on-screen hit me hard, and I felt my eyes filling with tears of relief.

Crucially, as the day went on, I started to remember small but increasingly clear details about myself and my family. Just the night before, when my nurse Nellie had asked me gentle questions about my boys, I'd become very distressed by not being able to remember the name of their school, or what year group they were in. Like with my coughing, I had a distorted perception that if I could answer these questions correctly, the medical staff would see that I was well enough to go home. It upset me hugely when I couldn't. Now however, little over twelve hours later, I was thrilled to realise I could actually remember the name of their school, as well as their ages - twelve and nine years old – and that they both loved maths, footy, and all things basketball! What incredible joy it brought me to remember these details of my boys! And that rainy Sunday, when I spoke to Matt, Jesaia and Coby on a video call my nurse set up on my phone, for the first time since waking from the coma the conversation felt light and filled with hope. I remember noticing that Jesaia and Coby were wearing jumpers, and asking if the weather outside was now cold. Over the screen my boys showed me the toys and games that loving family and friends had dropped off at the front door for them, and talking about the gifts provided Jesaia and Coby with a welcome distraction from seeing the tubes that still ran out of my neck and arms. The morning before, Saturday, I'd had my first video call with my boys since waking from the coma, eight days after they'd last seen me. This was the call that Matt described in his journal as making me very emotional, although I remember very little about the conversation. One thing I can picture very clearly however, is the intense look of upset - almost fear - on Coby's face as he saw me still clearly unwell, confused and disoriented. I was so far from the smiling, easy-speaking mother he was used to, and he struggled to keep looking at me through the phone, obviously deeply unsettled by the tubes and my robotic voice. Matt had to gently encourage Coby to speak to me, but he found it very difficult to know what to say. Now however, just a day later, the darkness had lifted, a sense of clarity was returning to my mind, and I delighted in talking more freely with Jesaia and Coby, who were full of stories about their new toys and books. When loving family and friends bought those gifts for our boys, they didn't just give them something to play with as a distraction while I was in the coma – they provided much-needed relief from the situation, which led to a connection over video call between two young boys and their mother, separated by 150 kilometres and an isolation room. I'll always remember and be so very grateful for that.

As the day went on, my nurse Georgia and I would talk about our dogs (I could now remember I had a dog! – gorgeous Indi, the gentle black greyhound), and watch *Escape to the Country* together on TV, pining after the green English countryside and choosing which house we would each pick. Such simple interactions brought me a huge amount of comfort and reassurance, and I could feel the anxiety and fear that had gripped me for two days continuing to lift.

And later that afternoon I would receive a very special surprise on my phone – a video my dear friend had taken that morning of our church community waving at the camera, some calling out words of encouragement and support, others praising God for my survival and healing. Georgia stood beside my bed holding my phone for me to see, and together we watched one masked face after the other fill the screen, lit up with those 'eye smiles'. It was a picture of God's family expressing His joy and love.

Let us love one another, for love comes from God. (1 John 4:7)

The evening of that Sunday marked a huge shift in my mental state, both medically and psychologically, as I approached my third night post-coma. When the evening nurse Jodie entered my ICU room to begin her twelve-hour shift, she immediately followed Georgia's cue by writing her name in black marker on the front of her disposable gown. Already the evening felt more settled and calmer, and I could feel the very tangible presence of God's peace over me. A monumental difference from the two previous nights was a noticeable improvement of the psychedelic swirls and flashes of colour that had caused me so much confusion and anxiety every time I closed my eyes. As the effects of the medication that had been holding me in the coma slowly relinquished their grip on my mind and body, the sheer relief I felt of being relieved of this distressing side effect was indescribable. Now my nurse Jodie turned her attention to my night ahead, concerned that I'd been without sleep for forty-eight hours straight now. Months later I would meet Professor Ed Litton from Fiona Stanley Hospital who, through his research, has addressed the detrimental effects of sleep deprivation on the recovery of ICU patients. Professor Litton says evidence shows that sleep quality in intensive care has a significant impact on the patient's health outcomes and recovery, both in hospital and post-discharge, and that simple acts such as routinely offering ear plugs to patients could reduce nighttime confusion and encourage deeper rest. And that's exactly what my efficient nurse Jodie did that night, hunting down a pair of earplugs (no small feat when leaving my isolation room meant complete removal of her PPE to avoid cross-contamination) and fashioning an eye-mask for me out of a flannel to reduce the amount of light that crept into my still-overstimulated mind. Another practical – and somewhat unusual! – action that Jodie took on my request was to stand on a chair to place a towel over a fixed clock on the wall of my room. As is common with many ICU patients – particularly those impacted by medication – time, and how fast it moved, had become a fixation for me. During those first distressing 48 hours after waking from the coma, my understanding of time had become severely warped, with every minute on the clock that I watched like a hawk feeling like an hour. When I literally couldn't move for all of the tubes, it made my severe claustrophobia even more pronounced – feeling bound both physically to my bed and in time by the clock. Once I became capable of speaking to Matt or my parents on the phone, it opened up a lifeline to my loved ones I so desperately craved, and again I became fixated on time. If Matt told me he'd call my phone again at 10am, I'd focus on the clock intently until that time arrived, and then become very distressed if the phone didn't ring exactly on the click of the hour. My world had become very insular and lacking in context – confined to the four walls of my isolation room – and so the details of what I could focus on became all-consuming. The clock and its ticking time had also taunted me for the past two nights as I lay awake unable to sleep, and so now Jodie stood on the chair trying multiple times to hang a towel over it to cover the face before finally having success – a task, she joked, that wasn't normally in her job description as a nurse!

And, finally, as I prepared myself my for another night of trying to sleep, Jodie asked if I'd like some soft music played in the darkness of the room, having learnt from my previous nurses how music had helped to calm me during my moments of confused distress. Ever since I'd woken from the coma, my nurses had been asking me simple questions each day about my life and loved ones, to gauge where my understanding was at and to encourage me to remember more details. That morning my nurse Georgia had commented on how gentle, supportive and loving Matt was on the phone every time we spoke, and asked how long we'd been married for. It wasn't easy to encourage my muddled brain to do the sums on that one, but eventually I established that in a couple of weeks' time we'd have been married for twenty years – not a bad effort considering I was only one year off the correct answer! At that stage I was still expected to be in hospital for many weeks yet, and so I became upset that I'd be spending our twentieth wedding anniversary recovering in Perth away from Matt and home. A phone call to Matt shortly after, however, reassured me that it was actually our nineteenth anniversary coming up! With my fixation on details at that point I was very relieved, especially when Matt promised me we would do something very special to celebrate our marriage when I came out of hospital. From that moment that promise became something on the 'outside' to look forward to and focus on, and so now when Jodie asked if I'd like gentle music played in my room as I tried to sleep, I asked for easy jazz – a favourite of mine which I often played in the background at home. And so I lay in my hospital bed wearing the flannel-made eye mask, thanking God for the incredible sense of relief from the psychedelic colours and explosions behind my eyes, and picturing the scene of a special anniversary dinner with my husband while jazz music played in the background. I'd like to be able to say I finally slept that night, but I didn't. However, a tangible sense of calm filled my mind and body, and for the first time in forty-eight hours I rested fully in His peace.

Chapter Fourteen

Just a few days before, Matt had been warned by my doctors that I'd likely remain in hospital for up to six weeks after coming off ECMO – one week for every day I'd spent on the life-support machine. And so it was now, on the Monday morning – less than three days after coming out of the coma – that I really began to understand the incredible reality of my medical recovery. During my week in the coma, and in the days since, the ICU Intensivist Dr Allen (he of the orange duck beak face mask) had come into my room daily. During each visit Dr Allen would perform an ultrasound on my heart, and now on this Monday morning he showed me the portable screen held in his hands, enthusiastically pointing to one of the veins. This vein, he explained, had swollen to three centimetres in diameter – double the normal size - when I was at my sickest on ECMO. Inflexible and inflated, it had been like a balloon ready to burst. Now, just days later, the vein had shrunk back to half its previous size, reducing to a healthy one and a half centimetres in width. Dr Allen also pointed out that the vein was now flexible and "wriggling like a worm", indicating healthy, consistent blood flow to the heart. Praise God! Meanwhile an artery, which had begun shriveling up due to a disruption in my blood supply from the cardiogenic shock, had now returned to normal as well, exciting Dr Allen in its speed of recovery. After being described as 'the sickest patient in ICU', with a heart so diseased it wasn't initially responding to medication or treatment on ECMO life support, I was now literally watching it heal before my very eyes. On an ultrasound screen held in the skilled hands of my doctor was the image of a heart that had been held in the healing hands of my Heavenly Protector.

That morning a physiotherapist also came into my room and helped me out of bed, the first time my feet had touched the ground in nine days. As I took a few very tentative steps away from my bed, with my nurse and the physiotherapist each firmly holding onto one of my arms to support me, I praised God with tears filling my eyes. Although I was still attached to a number of tubes in my neck and wrists, I felt intense relief at finally being upright and out of my hospital bed. While I'd been in the coma my body had built up almost ten kilograms of fluid, which was now gradually reducing due to medication. On that morning my feet were still puffy and swollen, and walking across the floor of my hospital room felt far from normal - a strange sensation as though I was stepping in water-filled gumboots. The physiotherapist reassured me that this was to be expected, and reminded me of just how far I'd come in such an incredibly short time. Just three days ago, my husband had been prepared that, despite me being taken off the life-support ECMO, I might still be in the induced coma and on the breathing machine for up to a week further – and yet here I was, awake, talking and now standing! Needless to say, Matt couldn't believe his eyes when my nurse rang him via video call and he saw me out of my hospital bed and sitting upright in a chair!

The physical healing of my heart and body was now astounding medical staff in its speed and strength. Almost every time a doctor or nurse would speak with me, or with Matt over the phone, they'd express their amazement at my "remarkable recovery", given how incredibly sick I'd been just days before. One nurse – who was called over from another section of the hospital on my final evening in ICU when my rostered night nurse became unwell – excitedly exclaimed "You're the ECMO lady!" when she realised who she'd be caring for. A number of nurses who'd cared for me while I was on ECMO at my most critically unwell - when my survival was far from guaranteed - would actually dress in PPE to be able to come into my room, wanting to see with their own eyes my rapid recovery post-coma. Some became quite emotional, and one nurse in particular had tears in her eyes as she shared with me that she'd been on shift when my friend rang through to my ICU room to pray over me as I lay in the coma. It was the first I knew this had happened, and I was incredibly moved to see how impacted she'd clearly been. During these visits, more than one nurse said to me "Someone was definitely watching out for you!" In those shared moments of wonder, I knew with full confidence exactly Who that Protecter and Healer was - and continued to be!

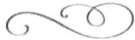

At the same time, however, my emotional struggle in still having not seen Matt and our boys since waking from the coma was intensifying. I was still testing positive to covid, and probably would do for quite some time, the doctors warned, due to my body being immuno-suppressed and therefore taking longer to shed the virus. And so while I remained in ICU, restrictions continued to prevent me from having my husband, children and parents by my bedside. Many months later, Matt and I would meet with and spend hours talking to the thoughtful and gracious ECMO specialist Dr Allen. We would share with him the significance of the huge emotional burden the restrictions had placed on the situation at the time, and the impact of Matt not having been allowed to be by my side, both during the coma and in my hospital recovery afterwards. Dr Allen quietly listened and shared his understanding, and then Matt asked him a question that I'll never forget, as it unveiled our lingering trauma from that time – "If it had become clear that Abbey wasn't going to survive the ECMO life support, would I have been allowed to visit her to see her before she died?" And the answer - delivered with much compassionate difficulty - was no. Under the restrictions at the time, it would not have been allowed.

And now, three days after waking from the coma, and ten days since I'd last seen my husband on that sidewalk outside Bunbury Hospital, the emotional impact of our enforced separation was increasingly taking its toll. My doctors were sympathetic and understanding of this, and recognised the need to balance the needs of my emotional health with my physical recovery. Crucially, Matt was now testing negative after his own ten days of covid, and so medical staff began trying to work out a way for him to visit me in ICU, although my isolation status in Pod Four made the situation very difficult.

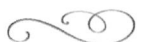

In so much of life it's often the little details that stick in our minds and have the most impact on us. I remember that Monday as the day two different doctors crouched down on their heels beside my hospital bed to lower themselves to my height as we talked. Such a simple yet intuitively caring and personable act, and one that touched me deeply after days of lying on my back in bed staring up at medical staff as they appeared to loom over me. The first doctor – a heart specialist I remember as Dr Brian – spoke gently and compassionately as he explained they were trying to work through all of the restrictions in bringing Matt in to see me but, if it happened, it would be my husband alone and not with our boys. After a number of phone calls were made that afternoon, it was organised that two of my doctors would meet with representatives from the hospital's Health Department the following day, Tuesday, to try to come to a solution that would enable me to finally see Matt. My health and recovery needed it, they agreed. And so with the prayerful hope that I would soon be reunited with part of my family for the first time since before the coma, I entered into my fifth evening without sleep. The second doctor to crouch down beside my bed, lowering himself to my eye level, arrived later that night, his voice full of warmth and compassion as he acknowledged my anxiety over my constant wakefulness. He agreed that five nights without sleep was not at all helpful to my recovery, and gave me some medication to calm my churning mind. Although it didn't give me the solid rest my body so desperately needed, I did sleep on and off for an hour at a time – which, in comparison to previous nights, felt like sweet relief.

Chapter Fifteen

Autumn. My absolute favourite time of year, especially the second half of the season. I love everything about it – the cooling temperatures that gradually bring about crisp, dewy mornings; the smells of wood fires and moist earth that begin to fill the air; the warmth of sunlight on the skin that feels healing and embracing rather than burning; the visual beauty of vibrant oranges, reds and yellows, as autumn trees prepare for the oncoming winter. Our family has a deciduous tree in our backyard that marks the passing of the seasons through its leaves, and noticing those first flashes of yellow and orange peeking through the post-summer abundance of green has always brought me such joy – as though autumn has quietly but confidently announced its arrival. In the days following the coma, my nurses would regularly question me on the day and date, to encourage the return of my memory. As I began to register that April was almost half over, I felt a growing sadness that I'd be spending my favourite season inside the walls of the hospital, confined to an intensive care unit while autumn marched on with its spectacular parade outside. On that Tuesday, Matt sent through to my phone a photo of the tree in our backyard, its leaves already displaying bright accents of yellow and orange that hadn't been apparent just two weeks earlier. Along with the photo, Matt wrote the simple message "You need to come home to see your tree". My heart ached to be home – with my family, my loved ones, my dog, my tree – and my tears fell easily in that moment. But, like the jazz music and promise of a special wedding anniversary celebration, the photo of the tree became an encouragement of hope of God's many blessings waiting for me on the outside.

Later in the morning on Tuesday came a very exciting development. An approved covid-isolation room had become available in the cardiology ward within the hospital, and my doctors were confident my recovery had been strong enough to transfer me across. This was incredible! Just days before I'd been in a critical condition on ECMO life support, and now I was being moved out of the intensive care unit weeks ahead of schedule. God's healing work was yet again on powerful display! Changing wards would also greatly increase the possibility of Matt being able to visit me for the first time, as we'd no longer be bound by the stricter protocols of the ICU. There was huge excitement as I spoke to Matt and our boys on the phone, with the day of finally being reunited as a family becoming closer.

It was now April twelfth, and Good Friday was just three days away. Another significant reason why I've always held a love for autumn is due to it being the season of Easter – by far my favourite celebration of the year. It's hard to put into words how deeply meaningful the event marking the crucifixion and resurrection of our Saviour Jesus Christ is to me. It's a time of deep reflection, intense gratitude, praise and worship, as I thank our God for His ultimate sacrifice. Our family always begins the Easter weekend with a moving service at our church, followed by a hot cross bun morning tea in our home filled with friends and fellowship. It's a tradition that started many years ago, as a way to invite into our home people who might not have family to spend the weekend with. It's now a time that we look forward to every year, with morning tea usually rolling into lunch and afternoon tea! Again, I felt a deep sadness that I wouldn't be at home to celebrate Easter with my precious family and friends, and so our attention turned towards enabling Matt to visit me for the first time in the cardiology unit on Good Friday. What an incredible day that would be!

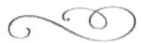

My nurse on that Tuesday was Grace, kind and gently spoken. Grace spent the majority of her shift preparing me for the move to the cardiology unit, as I tried to comprehend finally leaving the room in which I'd woken from the coma. As much as it had confined me and distorted my reality for the past four days, the space was all I'd known since coming off life support. Late that afternoon my bed on wheels was pushed through the door of my ICU room and out into the corridor, and I could now see the space where, only four nights earlier, I'd frantically believed people were being chased and attacked. Those forms now took shape as doctors, nurses and other medical staff, who were walking past or gathered in the nursing station which was directly outside my room. With my bed being pushed down the corridor, my head swivelled from side to side as I tried to take in everything from my surroundings. Many staff were still covered in PPE, but others wore just a face mask and, in contrast, the humanness of their appearance brought a sudden rush of tears to my eyes. Out of the confines of a single room, I now tried to make sense of where I was in the hospital, wondering if this was the same hallway I'd been urgently carried through in such a critical condition ten days earlier. Having never been inside Fiona Stanley Hospital before nothing looked familiar, but the sensation of finally being amongst people, movement, talking and general hospital activity was so incredibly reassuring.

As much as I'd spent the past four days longing to be released from the confines of my ICU room, I struggled to adjust to my new space in the cardiology ward that night. I'd become used to having a nurse with me in my room twenty-four hours a day and their constant presence had brought me a huge amount of comfort, especially when I was missing my family so much. Now in cardiology, I was also in an isolation room but without the permanent extra human of the ICU. Instead, medical staff in face masks – but now thankfully without the full PPE - would check on me regularly, and I was told I could call one of the nurses using the phone in my room if I needed help at any time. The other big change in my surroundings was the inclusion of a bathroom with toilet and shower. During the coma and in ICU a catheter had been inserted, along with the many other tubes running into me. The nurses had also given me a sponge bath in bed every day, with my Monday night nurse spending much of the evening carefully washing, drying and braiding my long hair – which lit up Matt's face with a huge smile when he saw the result over our nighttime video call! Now in cardiology, it was a big adjustment to take myself to the bathroom, spending over an hour that night slowly and painfully moving through the shower and then re-dressing. It was at this point I realised how intensely bruised my body was from the many tubes and injections

I'd had in my mid-section – my skin was completely covered in a deep purple and black colour from the tops of my thighs to below my rib cage, and it was a huge shock to see. When I finally made it back to my bed I spoke to Matt and our boys on my phone, yet again longing to hear their loving voices in person rather than from so far away. The nursing station was directly outside the internal window of my room, and so the softly chattering voices of the staff were a comfort to me that night as I tried to rest, acutely aware that I was alone in my hospital room for the first time since waking from the coma. With sleep refusing to come yet again, and a now-familiar physical ache of loneliness in my chest, I lay in the darkness focusing my thoughts on God's faithful promise that He is always with us – wherever we are, whatever the circumstances. The ache remained, but peace was restored, and I finally slept.

Yet I am not alone, for my Father is with me. (John 16: 32)

Chapter Sixteen

My care had now been transferred from the ICU doctors to cardiologist Dr Felicity Lee, who came into my room on Wednesday morning to examine me. Dr Lee's face was mostly hidden by a surgical mask, but I could hear the kindness in her voice as she spoke to me about the past two weeks and my separation from my family, quietly sympathetic of my desperate need to see them for the first time post-coma. Just as the ECMO specialist had done every day in ICU, Dr Lee now performed another ultrasound in my room, voicing her amazement at the strength and speed of my heart's recovery. The left ventricle was now functioning at sixty-seven percent, classified in the normal range of blood output – a phenomenal healing of a 'nonfunctional heart' that had been pumping at less than ten percent when I was flown to Perth. I had been so critically unwell for six days on life-support and yet now, based on my incredibly strong recovery Dr Lee could see happening before our very eyes, she was already quietly confident that I'd have no long-term effects from the near-fatal cardiogenic shock. Given there had been so many life-threatening risks during my illness, both in the days before and during the coma, God's hands had truly performed a miracle in fully healing and restoring my diseased and failing heart, and protecting the rest of my body from serious and long-term harm. I couldn't praise Him enough.

That afternoon as I was again alone in my room, I sat in a chair by the shuttered, firmly sealed window, a Bible resting in my lap. My sister and brother-in-law had just dropped off a care package to the hospital's reception containing the Bible as well as ear plugs, an eye mask (a proper one, not a flannel!), lip balm, new underwear, a book and chocolate – all the essentials for a long-term hospital stay. Reading God's Word and His faithful promises had brought me strength and encouragement, and I now turned to watch through the window as people walked and cycled along the street below in the mid-April sunshine. In that moment my yearning to be free of the four walls of my isolation room – to feel fresh air on my face and sunlight on my skin – intensified, and I vowed never again to take for granted the gift of physical freedom, movement and a healthy body. A vow that could easily be forgotten when life returned to a sense of normality. But to this day, when I take in the river or bush during my daily five kilometre walk, I remember that window-side chair in the corner of my hospital room, and I praise God for every step forward I'm taking.

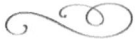

"We think you'll be able to go home tomorrow".

I don't think I could have been more shocked by a sentence than I was in that moment. It was later on that Wednesday afternoon, and Dr Lee had returned to my room for another examination. Only hours before my sister had delivered to the hospital the extra supplies, in readiness of my extended stay in the cardiology ward. And yet now Dr Lee was looking at me with smiling eyes, telling me I could be home in time for Easter! In that moment it almost became too much for my thoughts and emotions to comprehend. My family hadn't seen me for twelve days, since before I'd been flown to Perth and placed on life support. I'd only been missing them for five days, but that time had felt like five years as I'd battled the post-coma traumas without them. Our focus over the past day had been to work out a way for Matt to spend Good Friday with me in my hospital room, and the thought of that reunion had been exhilarating. But now I was being told I might be going home! – to spend Easter in the embrace of my family where I ached to be. Dr Lee warned me there were a few crucial requirements to meet before it became a reality though. I still had extensive bruising from the many injections and tubes placed into my body, especially over my thighs and lower torso, and across my groin area, which would need to be examined with ultrasound to make sure there was no internal damage. Most of the many tubes' entry points into my body – through my neck, wrists and legs – had already begun to heal very well, but I did have two large wounds just below the right side of my groin that needed ongoing care. This upper part of my leg was where the two largest tubes had been surgically inserted into my body and directed to my heart, attaching me to the ECMO machine as it pumped my freshly oxygenated blood back into my arteries. Given that one of these tubes had been the width of an adult's thumb, the wounds they'd left in my groin were significant and would take quite some time to heal. They needed to be drained regularly, and cleaned and re-dressed daily, and incredibly this now seemed to be a greater concern in sending me home than my rapidly-healing heart was!

The other concern was that, living 150 kilometres away from the hospital, I wouldn't be close by, should anything with my recovery go wrong. Now that the idea of going home to my family tomorrow had been planted I couldn't focus on any other alternative, and so I told Dr Lee I'd be more than willing to travel the one and half hours back to Fiona Stanley Hospital as often as needed for check-ups. Dr Lee was still clearly hesitant about this, but when a medical plan emerged to have me visit Bunbury Hospital daily to have my recovery monitored and my wounds cleaned and dressed, possibility started to become reality! It was decided I'd have another echocardiogram on my heart and ultrasound on my groin area the following morning, and if the cardiologist was satisfied with the results, I'd be given the go-ahead to leave hospital. The phone call to Matt and our boys, and then another to my parents, to share the news that I might be coming home tomorrow was met with disbelief and then tears of joy and excitement. Matt had now gone from anxiously waiting to hear if he could drive up to Perth on Good Friday to visit me for the first time, to being told he might be making the trip a day earlier to bring his wife home!

That evening as I lay in my hospital bed for what I prayed was the final night, I opened the Bible my sister had delivered to the hospital a day earlier. Matt had just sent me a text, encouraging me to read Psalm 30, and as the words of King David – written as a song of thanks to God for His healing mercy three thousand years ago – poured over me, my newly-healed heart began to hammer in my chest.

O Lord my God, I called to you for help and you healed me.
O Lord, you brought me up from the grave, you spared me from going down into the pit.

Sing to the Lord, you saints of his, praise his holy name.
For his anger lasts only a moment, but his favour lasts a lifetime.
Weeping may remain for a night, but rejoicing comes in the morning.
When I felt secure I said, "I will never be shaken."
O Lord, when you favoured me, you made my mountain stand firm;
But when you hid your face, I was dismayed.
To you, O Lord, I called,
To the Lord I cried for mercy:
"What gain is there in my destruction, in my going down into the pit?
Will the dust praise you?
Will it proclaim your faithfulness?
Hear, O Lord, and be merciful to me.
O Lord be my help."
You turned my wailing into dancing,
You removed my sackcloth and clothed me with joy,
That my heart may sing to you and not be silent.
O Lord my God, I will give you thanks forever. (Psalm 30:2-12)

King David's song of praise to God after his healing from a serious illness perfectly described the stages of my own life-threatening battle over the past two weeks. My time of stillness in the coma... the nights of weeping tears… the many prayers on my behalf for mercy and healing… being restored from a place close to death… praise and celebration… the darkness of the days to follow… the ongoing healing of my mind, body and heart. In that moment I knew with all certainty that the One who'd brought me up from the grave was asking me – commanding me! – to forever sing His praises for what He'd done, to boldly tell others of his miraculous works and faithfulness. It was still very early days in my journey of illness and recovery, but God was already showing me that, through Him, good would pour out of the traumatic events of the past two weeks, and it would begin with glorifying His powerful name. In that moment, for the first time I truly began to understand the full extent of God's healing mercy and, lying in my hospital bed, I began to weep tears of humility and gratitude. Just as King David had declared thousands of years earlier, my vow as I now prepared to return home was a heart that would not stay silent in singing the praises of its Almighty Healer.

Chapter Seventeen

"I'm not religious, but I just wanted to tell you that I think someone must have been looking out for you".

I'd heard words to this effect a number of times over the past week, and now as I was sitting upright on the end of my hospital bed waiting to be released into the eager arms of my family, they were spoken to me again.

It was mid-afternoon on Thursday, one day before Good Friday, and exactly two weeks since my heart had begun its descent into cardiogenic shock. For the first time since then I was out of my hospital gown and compression socks and wearing regular clothes and shoes. I'd re-entered my room after very slowly showering and dressing that morning to find four medical staff patiently waiting for me, each ready to begin their separate tests and scans that would determine if I was actually going home. It still seemed too amazing to be true – but then, how could I possibly be surprised by anything in God's power after the events of the past two weeks? The first ultrasound of the day showed a heart that was continuing its solid recovery, the reassuring sound of a strong, healthy heartbeat filling the room. Blood tests results were also pleasing to the cardiologist, showing that a number of markers indicating the severity of my heart failure had now significantly reduced. The second scan, this time of my groin area where the two largest tubes had been inserted, was undertaken on the lower ground floor of the hospital, requiring my bed to be pushed through multiple corridors and into an elevator. Crucially, this ultrasound confirmed no internal damage, despite the extensive bruising and firmness of the area. Returned to my room, I sat up in bed trying to read a book, but my thoughts were firmly focused on how close I was to finally seeing my family again. As it turned out my first sight of them came less than an hour later, through the window of my third-floor room as they stood on the grass verge across the road below. Matt had been told by nursing staff over the phone that I probably wouldn't be released until mid-afternoon, but he, Jesaia and Coby had arrived in Perth by late morning, determined to be ready and waiting for the moment I left hospital. Because I had no bearings as to where my cardiology room was positioned within the extensive hospital layout, I wasn't able to guide Matt and our boys to the direction of my window. And so a phone call from Matt to let me know they'd arrived in Perth and were now sitting on a patch of lawn near a small lake opposite the hospital to eat their lunch was met with huge excitement when I realised that exact location was directly underneath my window! I climbed out of bed as quickly as I could and made my way across the room, my heart hammering as I saw my family on the verge below, anxiously peering up to scan the multitude of hospital windows for the first sight of their wife and mother. From their viewpoint on the ground I was little more than a shadowy figure standing in the window, and it took a moment for them to be sure it was me. But as I stood on the other side of the glass waving frantically, tears rolling down my cheeks, Matt's face lit up with joy and Jesaia and Coby began jumping around with excitement. Now the closest we'd been to each other in two weeks – with just a pane of glass and fifty metres separating us – we spent the next hour talking on the phone while the boys played football on the grass below, often asking "Mum, can you see my next kick?" while looking up at my window to make sure I was still there watching. They definitely didn't need to check though – in that moment, nothing could have torn my eyes away from the sight of my family! Eventually I did have to turn away when a nurse came into my room for a number of final checks, and Matt used that time to gather our boys in preparation for moving across to the hospital's entrance. With our reunion now tantalisingly close, I sat on the end of my bed with my small bag packed at my feet, ready for the hospital porter's arrival with a wheelchair to take me to my waiting family. It was now that I heard the words, "I'm not religious, but I just wanted to tell you that I think someone must have been looking out for you" – spoken to me by a nurse who'd just started her shift for the evening. I wasn't familiar with the gentle-sounding young woman, as she hadn't been one of the nurses who'd taken care of me over the past two days in the cardiology ward. But she was clearly aware of my illness and time spent on the ECMO life-support, and had now made the effort to come into my room before I left the hospital to express her relief and amazement at my recovery. With King David's words of praise *"My heart may sing to you and not be silent"* pressed upon my own thankful heart, I shared of the Almighty Someone who'd heard the faithful prayers of so many, and in His grace and mercy had healed me.

The distinctive squeaking sound of a wheelchair being pushed down the corridor outside my room signalled that my departure from the hospital was now only moments away, and my hands started shaking in anticipation. Seconds later the door to my room opened and a masked porter appeared, ready to transfer me downstairs to my waiting family. "You'll need to wear a mask too, you're heading through the main hospital now", the cardiology nurse said to me, and it was then I was hit by the full realisation that I was truly re-entering the world outside the four walls of my isolation bubble. The nurse gently helped me into the wheelchair and said a sincere goodbye, and the porter carefully pushed me down the corridor and into the elevator. Watching the numbers light up on the wall of the lift as we descended through the floors of the hospital, I warned the porter to brace himself for a lot of tears as he delivered me to my family. "Husband a bit of a softie at heart, is he?" he laughed, but then I watched the lighthearted expression in his eyes change to shock as I told him I'd been in hospital on ECMO life support, and restrictions meant I hadn't been allowed to see my family since being placed in a coma two weeks earlier. I was very moved to see the porter's eyes fill with tears as he quietly said "I'm so sorry to hear that. I can't imagine how your husband's been coping all this time". At that moment the elevator doors opened and we entered the hospital's foyer, my eyes adjusting to the natural light that seemed to pour in through the floor-to-ceiling windows. "Not long now" the porter murmured as we moved towards the hospital's entrance, and I felt my body begin to shake all over in nervous anticipation of the reunion to come. Seconds later the doors were opening for us, and the porter wheeled me out into the cool late afternoon April air – an instant shock to my skin after the climate-controlled confines of the past two weeks. "I think I know who your husband is" the porter said gently, and I followed the direction of his eyes to see Matt standing next to Jesaia and Coby by our parked car, tears rolling down his face. My husband was openly experiencing the intense emotion of this full-circle moment. I'd been taken away from him two weeks earlier in a wheelchair, as he watched helplessly from the pavement outside Bunbury hospital. And now here we were again, outside a hospital with me being pushed in a wheelchair – but this time, by the grace of God, I was moving *towards* him.

Jill's journal – Thursday 14th April, evening

You are home!! It has been a long, agonising, prayer-filled, fearful, despairing – and then overwhelmingly joyful – fourteen days. We have intensely suffered over you nearly dying several times... and then your body steadied... and then you miraculously came back to us in a completely incomprehensible and amazing way. Incomprehensible, maybe... except that we were given assurance time and again, even in the darkest hours, that you were in the strong arms of the Almighty God of Heaven. You were also attended minute by minute by skilled doctors and nurses, who made wise and brave decisions concerning your heart and well-being. We prayed for God to guide their hands and decision-making as they worked tirelessly to keep you alive, and then help you on your healing pathway. We continue to thank God for them, and give all praise and worship to our Miracle Worker!!

Chapter Eighteen

Drive-through coffee. Drive-through fast food. Drive-through liquor stores. Even drive-through chemists. We're a society that loves the convenience of not having to get out of our cars while picking up supplies or running errands. Never before though had I encountered a drive-through medical examination. Another moment on that Friday to add to my ever-growing list of surreal experiences over the past fortnight.

But first, breakfast.

It was Good Friday, the morning after I'd been reunited with my family and arrived home from hospital. What had always been a day of deep gratitude and reflection now came with an intensely emotional layer – our Almighty God had offered new life through the death and resurrection of His only Son two thousand years ago, and now He'd physically saved my life again. It wasn't yet 9am, but the tears had already spilled.

I sat in our back patio, my senses soaking in the sights, smells and sounds I'd craved while in hospital isolation – the crispness of the mid-April morning air on my skin, the light mist that settled over the trees in the near distance, the twittering chatter of two small birds dancing on our fence. In front of me sat a plate of sourdough toast, piled high with scrambled eggs, smoked salmon, avocado and rocket leaves. My clear memory of that breakfast remains in my mind (and tastebuds) to this day! Due to the daily impact of a decades-long battle with inflammatory bowel disease I followed a low-FODMAP diet, which restricted or eliminated a number of foods that had proven to cause me cramping, inflammation and pain after eating. Ironically, onion and garlic – considered to be 'superfoods' for their health-protective benefits – are two of those foods for me. It can often feel overwhelming to prepare food for a person on the low-FODMAP diet – my own mum will comfortably admit she's mastered a handful of recipes to cook for me and won't deviate from those! Add to the mix a busy hospital kitchen with limited time or means to cater for varying food requirements and, when I was able to slowly start eating again in ICU, I found myself being served the same two meals every day - gluten-free cornflakes in a sugarcane bowl (fully disposable, as most items leaving my isolation room were required to be) for breakfast, and baked chicken with carrots and potatoes (no gravy, due to those sneaky onion and garlic powders) for both lunch and dinner. Although incredibly thankful for mouthfuls of food that came without tubes or nausea, I soon started to feel less than excited at the sight of potatoes, and began craving a meal that would provide a nutritious kickstart to both my body and the day. And so now, as I ate my first post-hospital breakfast with not a sugarcane bowl or bamboo spoon in sight, I savoured every delicious, flavoursome mouthful. I still rate it one of the best meals I've ever had!

Following that glorious breakfast was another emotional reunion – this time with my parents, who'd been holding off impatiently from driving to our house first thing that morning! Just like the day before with Matt and our boys, the tears flowed freely and the hugs were long, saved up over two weeks of life-changing separation. Then it was time to leave again – my parents would now stay with Jesaia and Coby at our home while Matt drove me to Bunbury Hospital so a nurse could check over the wounds in my groin area. I can't actually recall why the examination became a drive-through one – I think it was probably a mix of reasons. It was the Good Friday public holiday, at the height of WA's reported covid case numbers (with a specialist drive-through covid clinic at Bunbury Hospital), and my doctors in Perth were hoping to restrict the number of times I had to enter the hospital due to my immunocompromised body. Either way, we arrived at the drop-off car bay outside the entrance to the hospital to find a nurse waiting for us, in the very same spot Matt had been forced to leave me exactly two weeks earlier. At this point I still remembered nothing of that frantic trip to hospital on April Fools' Day, and so being back there felt strange and unsettling – having known intellectually what had happened – but didn't bring on any sensations of panic. That would come later. It did shake Matt up however, as memories of watching me being wheeled away from him came flooding back. This time I was staying put though, seated in the passenger side of the car as the masked nurse leant in through the window with more of those eye smiles, introducing herself and explaining what she needed to examine – the wounds in my groin area, the dressing and drainage tube covering them, and the heavy black bruising that extended from my upper thighs to my midsection. By now I was well and truly used to having my body poked and prodded after almost two weeks in ICU, and so the in-car examination didn't seem as strange as it probably should have. Eventually given the all-clear and instructed to return to the same place the next day for round two of checks, Matt again drove away from Bunbury Hospital on a Friday – but this time, I was coming home with him.

Easter Sunday. The King is risen! Early morning cloud gave way to a blue sky and gentle sunshine, and when Matt asked how I'd like to celebrate that special day, I knew instantly. My parents owned two acres of land about fifteen minutes' drive from our house, thick with bush and overlooking the paddocks of neighbouring farmland. It was secluded, tranquil and the perfect spot for a simple morning tea. At the top of a hill, which opened to a clearing surrounded by trees, stood a large, rustic wooden cross, placed there by the local church a number of years ago for their dawn Good Friday service. It had always been a powerful and moving sight, especially in the early-morning mist. On this day, Matt drove our car as far as he could take it on the track up the hill. He and my parents then carefully helped me out of the car, and we very slowly walked the rest of the way to the top. My dad was the first to start crying, and I was smiling through my own tears – still so weakened but exhilarated by the moment of being alive in God's creation on this Easter Sunday. Despite Matt and my dad each holding one of my arms, I was physically exhausted by the short walk to the area my mum had set up for our morning tea, and gratefully sank into a chair placed there for me. Together as a family we sang and prayed, an outpouring of praise and worship for all our Saviour had done – and continued to do. I closed my eyes and let the words wash over me, my tears expressing my overwhelming gratitude of being alive in that moment. Later, after morning tea, my mum hid clues on slips of paper throughout the bush, leading Jesaia and Coby to a final stash of chocolate eggs – an activity I've always found such joy in doing with the children in my life. I cried again, overcome with emotion at seeing the looks of excitement on my boys' faces as they tore through the bush in search of the next clue. I returned home to rest shortly after, my fragile body exhausted by the simple outing, my heart filled with gratitude and wonder at being able to spend this precious day with my family in this way, when I should have still been in hospital.

For as long as I live, I'll never forget that victorious Easter Sunday.

God set him free from death and raised him to life. Death could not hold him in its power (Acts 2:24) CEV

Chapter Nineteen

I had questions that desperately needed answering. So many questions.

In the days spent in ICU following my time on ECMO, I'd heard over and again how critically unwell I'd been over the past week. I knew I'd been in a coma, and I was starting to slowly understand just how many people around the world had been praying for my survival. But I knew very little of any actual details. The strengthening and recovery of my severely damaged heart was the main focus of my medical team, who often said to me during my time in ICU, "Your priority now is to stay calm and restful for your recovering heart".

It was now Monday afternoon, and I'd been home from hospital for almost four days. During that time I'd received a number of phone calls from loving family and friends. The calls didn't last long, as I was still very weakened and tired, unable to talk for more than five or ten minutes at the most. Each time, the person on the other end was joyous over my recovery and return home, but also clearly hesitant as to how much they could talk to me about what had actually happened. And so on that

Monday my parents arrived at our house mid-afternoon, Matt prepared cups of tea, and we sat outside in the patio. My dad and mum carried worried expressions on their faces, concerned and hesitant about the conversation to come, and it suddenly hit me how utterly exhausted they looked after the events of the past few weeks.

As we sipped our tea – with me still relishing the warmth and taste of a simple English Breakfast in a non-disposable mug – Matt and my parents began to talk, carefully and gently, with many pauses to collect both their thoughts and emotions. They started with the phone call to the doctor in the early hours of that April Fools' Day, the panic Matt had felt as he drove me to Bunbury Hospital, the way my dad had been forced to sit in his car in our driveway to watch over his two young grandsons as they isolated inside. Tears filled Matt's eyes as he recalled his helplessness in watching medical staff wheel me away, and his frustration at not being able to help me inside the hospital. He and my parents talked me through their limited understanding of the events of that Friday night and the following Saturday morning, expressing their still-obvious confusion over the way the situation had escalated so rapidly. My parents' tears flowed easily, and I noticed my dad's hands shaking as they described to me the hours they'd spent waiting outside the hospital by the ambulance bay, hoping for a glimpse of their daughter before I was flown to Perth. "It was a warm day, and we were so thirsty as we'd left our water bottles in the car. But I didn't want to run back to get them, because I was scared they'd wheel you out at that exact time and I'd miss you". I could feel the pain of the moment in my mum's words, and my heart ached over the intense confusion they must have felt. My mum continued, "A nurse finally took us inside the hospital for something to drink and eat, and afterwards we realised they'd deliberately removed us from where we'd been waiting so we wouldn't see you in the state you were in when they loaded you into the ambulance". When an ICU consultant came into the family lounge to speak with my parents she confirmed this by admitting "It's the dads we always need to be careful with", sharing that the response by a father to seeing his daughter in grave danger is often the most emotional and potentially disruptive. My dad then picked up the story, telling me "The doctor was compassionate but she was also brutally honest, telling us that you were in a very bad way and it wasn't a certainty that you'd even survive the flight to Perth, even though they were doing everything they could. She said that because you're only forty-one, they'd consider every option available to keep you alive".

I've thought about those words a lot since then, and thanked God over and again for the blessing of my age and the healthy strength of my heart before I became unwell. One of the sensitive considerations that impacts decision-making when it comes to choosing which critically ill patients are placed on ECMO is the actual likelihood of them getting better on the life support. The survival rate of adults on ECMO is, on average, around fifty percent, with that figure dropping for patients aged over sixty-five. An international study which explored the use of ECMO for critically ill patients with covid found that those treated later in the pandemic were staying on the life support machine longer, and dying more often. The reality is, ECMO is a high-risk procedure that is very labour intensive, requiring highly trained and experienced medical staff with specialist skills – and so having patients stay on ECMO for a longer time utilises many resources and can lead to an increase in the likelihood of death. The urgency that Matt and my parents felt as each new day began and my critically diseased heart remained 'stable' but not adequately improving on the ECMO treatment was therefore very real. (That's another thing my Mum has talked about – coming to the harsh realisation that, when the ICU medical staff described my critically ill condition in the induced coma as 'stable', the term could lead to a false sense of security of how sick I still was. My mum explained, "I think I probably clung onto that word a lot. In the early days you were in the coma, my mind and heart were centred on "stable, stable, stable", convinced that meant your health would change for the better soon. On the Tuesday night, when another doctor gave Matt a very brutal assessment of your health and chances of living, despite your condition remaining – that word again - stable, this false sense of security came crashing down around me, and I quickly became very, very afraid. But God saw my confusion and fear, and He sent those three wonderful women to support me the next day when I 'crashed'. After that, our growing understanding of your dire condition matured, but so did our trust in God's direct hand over the situation.")

During our time sitting in the patio that Monday afternoon, Matt also described the moment he'd answered a phone call from a friend of ours as he and our boys had waited in the backyard to watch my RFDS plane fly overhead enroute to Perth. It was around 11.30am on the Saturday, with my parents still waiting outside Bunbury Hospital, and Matt yet to know that my flight had been delayed because of my deteriorating condition. Our friend, who works in pathology, had been on shift when the results from my overnight blood tests landed on his desk. Shocked by the dangerously high reading of troponin levels (indicating acute heart failure), he was – he much later admitted to me – fearful of my chances of survival. He rang Matt, not actually expecting him to answer the phone, but when they did connect and talked for a few minutes, our friend was hit with the realisation that Matt still had a limited understanding of exactly how potentially fatal the circumstances were. The situation was rapidly unfolding in uncertainty and confusion, with doctors at the hospital working hard to stabilise me, and Matt confined to our home and unable to know the full extent of my condition. Ever the professional, and respecting the ethics of his position, our friend didn't reveal any information to Matt, but instead offered his support and began praying in earnest as soon as he got off the phone. Yet another faithful prayer warrior whose position God utilised for good in that moment.

As the afternoon moved on, we shared more tea and tears as Matt and my parents tried to wade through the traumatic circumstances of my time in the coma on ECMO, constantly weighing up which details to include and what to leave out for another time. I was desperate to learn more, to fill in the huge gaps in my limited understanding of what had actually happened. To me, it felt very much like a terrible story that had happened to someone else – unable to remember anything about my time in Bunbury Hospital or being flown to Perth and then put on life support meant I was yet to form any kind of mental or emotional attachment to the events of that week. But it was still so incredibly real and raw for Matt and my parents, who were also very aware and protective of placing any further stress on my recovering heart. When Matt explained how an ICU consultant had phoned him from the hospital to say they were now preparing to put me on ECMO life support, he didn't choose this Monday outside in the patio to reveal his intense moment of distress when he was told he couldn't speak to me before I was placed in the induced coma. He would share that with me many months later – how he'd fell to the floor sobbing, pouring out to God his desperation to talk to me for even just a few short minutes. Our loving Father heard the cries of His child, and half an hour later I had stabilised enough to speak those precious words with Matt and our boys for the final time before slipping into unconsciousness.

Now, on this Monday in the patio, as my parents explained a little more to me about the life-threatening risks involved in putting me on ECMO, they admitted to not yet allowing themselves to see the photos of me surrounded by tubes and wires while attached to the life support machine that had been sent to Matt's phone by a nurse on my second day in the coma. Even in the safe assurance that I was now home with my family, finally able to be hugged and held, it would be many more weeks before they could bring themselves to see those images.

One thing that stands out to me from that Monday is learning that I'd faced the risk of possible limb amputation, had serious complications arisen from spending a longer time on the ECMO machine. More than any of the other risk factors being explained to me, that one hit the hardest. As an active and outdoors-loving woman, wife and mum of two playful, sporty young boys, I was suddenly overwhelmed by the realisation of how incredibly different my return home from hospital might have been. While all of the serious risks of ECMO can prove to be life-threatening or life-changing, this one impacted me the most, and in that moment I became very aware of the ongoing pain in my legs caused by the surgeries, tubes and wounds – and so intensely grateful to feel those sensations because it meant my legs were *there*.

But now the exhaustion was taking hold as I started to feel increasingly overwhelmed by the very details I was pushing to discover. And so Matt and my parents ended our emotional conversation that Easter Monday by sharing more with me of the incredible prayer chain that had grown from the afternoon I was flown to Perth and placed on life-support, and taken hold to become a powerful movement of God's people literally around the world. Prayer that covered my flight and road journey to hospital by ambulance. Prayer for the medical staff who would receive and assess me when I arrived in Perth. Prayer over rapid decision-making, treatment options and surgical hands. Prayer for comfort and strength for my family who were distressed, helpless and unable to be with me. Prayer over my unconscious body as I lay in the coma - pushing back against death, against medical odds, against anything other than whole and complete healing. In that moment I couldn't comprehend the enormity of it – and some days I'm still emotionally overwhelmed by the sense of humility and gratitude I feel. Many, many more stories of prayer would emerge in the months to come, including from people who shared it had been their first time of praying. God's children crying out to their Father in urgency, trust, faith and praise.

And then – again – I rested in Him.

Text message of gratitude – sent Tuesday 19th April
To the dear, precious people who prayed faithfully to our almighty God on my behalf – I love you all, and can't even begin to describe my overwhelming gratitude for the army of prayers that were spoken and cried. Coming home from hospital has been incredibly emotional for my family and me, a mix of pure joy and trauma. Absolute joy at God's miracle of healing. The doctors told Matt that complications with my organs could start if I was on the ECMO life support machine for more than three days, but I came off it after six days with none of those complications having happened. They told Matt that for every day I was in the coma I would need a week of recovery in hospital afterwards, but instead I spent one week recovering in

ICU and cardiology after being in the coma for six days. I had ICU doctors telling me every day they were amazed by the progress of my heart's recovery after how severe my heart failure (diagnosed as cardiogenic shock) was, and nurses saying to me "Someone was looking out for you". I'm still emotionally wrapping my head around the enormity of God's miracle, as there's a lot of details I'm still finding out slowly from Matt, my parents and the cardiologist about exactly how sick I was. Emotionally, Matt and I are very much feeling the trauma of not being able to have seen each other during those two weeks, especially for him while I was on life support, and for me when I came off it still so unwell with no idea what had happened over the past eight days. But the same God of miracles is holding our hands as we work through that slowly over time. Physically I have a lot of bruising from being on the ECMO machine, I still feel very weak and it will take time for my heart to strengthen, but the cardiologist says the outlook is very good, praise God. I love you all, and will forever be thankful for your faithful prayers to the Almighty One who saved my life. With all my love, Abbey.

I will walk humbly all my years because of this anguish... You restored me to health and let me live. (Isaiah 38:15...16)

Chapter Twenty

The sunshine was healing that autumn. In the weeks after returning home from hospital I spent hours each day sitting in our backyard, face often turned to the sky, soaking in the gentle warmth of the sun. Visitors came – hesitant and nervous at first seeing me, then open with hugs and tears. Hands were held, cups of tea drunk, books read. Many ongoing questions – continuing to piece together all that had happened – were asked in that warming sunshine. It was where Matt and I sat together on our nineteenth wedding anniversary, eating a cooked lunch lovingly prepared by my aunty. That was also the day Matt gave me the journal he'd kept while I was in hospital – the gift of a husband's unfaltering love and commitment. I hadn't known about Matt's daily writing – initially started as an attempt to keep track of the stream of medical information, machines, processes and names of doctors and nurses that poured over the phone each day, but which soon became a vital source of mental relief in his confusion and distress. A lot of Matt's writing, he told me, was done later at nighttime after our boys had gone to sleep – a much-needed release of thoughts, questions and emotions which had built up throughout the day. And now he was giving me this most precious and vulnerable of gifts on our anniversary, with the wise encouragement to take my time reading it at a pace that my emotions could handle. The next day, in that same warming sunshine, I began to read my husband's written words. Starting from the day I was taken to Bunbury Hospital, and moving through two weeks until I came home from Perth, Matt's daily journal entries painted an honest and emotional picture of a distraught family who didn't stop trusting and never gave up hope. He detailed the many phone conversations with nurses and doctors – describing surgeries, scenarios and decision-making that he could only be a part of from afar, and that I'll never remember. He wrote of the absolute necessity of the power of prayer from so many to carry him, our children and my parents through that week, day after day, and the practical love showered over our family. He shared of caring for our two young boys – who needed their father in a way they'd never experienced before – and remaining consistent and strong for them in those days of distressing confusion and uncertainty. I read most of Matt's words through a watery film – tears constantly filling my eyes, at times spilling over in a heave of sobbing. Now I understood why Matt had cautioned me to take my time in reading the journal, ever cautious of my ongoing recovery. My heart felt as though it was physically aching (words I don't write lightly, given what it had just been through) with love and emotion while reading Matt's honest outpouring of words. The gratitude and respect I felt for him as a husband, father and son-in-law was forceful, and I was in awe of the humility in his unwavering faith during some incredibly dark moments in that week of the life-support. Matt, by his own ready admission, is not a writer, has never been a journaller – and yet his faithful commitment to chronicling those deeply honest memories, thoughts, questions and prayers became a precious gift, and an integral part of this book.

Matt's final journal entry – written ten days after I came home from hospital

I can't express in words how relieved, grateful and happy I am that God has healed you and brought you home safely to our family! I will never again doubt God's love and faithfulness, and will forever be full of praise to Him. I experienced some very dark thoughts while you were on life support, wondering how I would get through life without you, and thinking that Jesaia and Coby were way too young to lose their mother. I questioned God as to why this was happening to you, but I never stopped trusting Him, praising Him or believing He would deliver you from this. Our Lord and Saviour sure is mighty to save! I was so determined that I would give you this journal once – not if – you were home recovered, and I'm so grateful I now can. You are such an amazingly strong and special woman who I'm so privileged to call my best friend and wife. This traumatic experience we've been through will only make our love for each other stronger. I just know that God will bring good out of this horrible time and use your testimony of healing to impact many people's lives and faith.

I love you so very much my dearest Abbey. With all my love forever, from your husband Matthew.

I also spent many afternoons in those early weeks lying quietly in bed, my aching, weakened and bruised body needing plenty of rest. Daytime naps have never come easily to me, and even now in my recovery I rarely slept during these times in bed. Instead, in the dark and cool of the room I'd have instrumental praise and worship music softly playing, and it would be a time of deep meditation on the Master Healer who'd never left my side. 'Way maker', 'Oceans', 'I Surrender', 'Still'… amongst the often chaotic confusion of my thoughts, questions and anxieties, the gentle music brought peace to my mind. Those hours spent lying in quiet communion with God each day – doing nothing other than focusing on the power of His saving grace – became an absolute necessity and, I strongly believe, an essential part of my recovery. I can truly say I've never felt closer or more connected to God than I did during those moments. As the weeks and then months went on, and I began to regain more strength, my afternoon rest times in the solitary peace of our quiet bedroom became gradually less frequent, and then eventually stopped altogether. At the time that was a cause for celebration – my recovery was strong, and I was welcoming the return of a more normal daily routine! It was some months later though, during conversation with a friend, that the realisation hit me of how much I missed – craved, in fact – those daily quiet, uninterrupted hours spent with God. The deep intimacy and understanding they'd brought, the gift of His soul-filling peace, as I'd meditated on nothing but His presence and goodness.

Chapter Twenty One

Mother's Day. Exactly one month since being taken off ECMO life support, and the day I would finally get to soak in those autumn colours I'd longed for while inside the restrictive walls of my isolation room. Apart from that precious Easter Sunday on my parents' bush block just days after being reunited with my family, the only times I'd left our home and its cocooning backyard were for my many appointments at the hospital, both in Bunbury and Perth, to undergo regular scans on my heart and have my wounds checked and dressed. Now we were heading to the Golden Valley Tree Park, a stunning arboretum nestled in the hills of Balingup, around an hour's drive from our house. Beautiful to visit all year round, the park truly stuns in autumn, with each tree jostling to outdo each other with vibrant bursts of red, yellow and orange. Matt and my mum had filled picnic baskets with my favourite foods (not a hospital-style boiled potato in sight!) and, with my parents following behind in their car, we headed south, winding our way through hills that weren't yet green after a particularly warm autumn. As if to prove the point, on this day we were all dressed in short sleeves, with Matt and our boys wearing shorts – no indication that winter was only three short weeks away. As Matt drove, I couldn't take my eyes off the scenery outside my open window, soaking in every detail, feeling like I was seeing God's creation through new eyes and fresh understanding. A cliché maybe, but truly the case. We pulled up in the arboretum's car park at the same time as my parents and, in a scene that mirrored Easter Sunday, Matt and my dad stayed close by my side as we walked over a small bridge and into the park together, heading for our favourite picnic spot under a towering flame tree. This time though as I walked I felt noticeably stronger, my legs able to cover more distance before the tiredness set in again. Working together around me (well, the adults at least – Jesaia and Coby had already run off to kick the footy!) my family set up chairs, spread out picnic rugs and loaded food onto tables in the shade of the tree. Before we ate my dad prayed, praising God for bringing me home to my husband and boys, for the gift of being here, on this special day of celebration, with my family. As we began to eat, I looked around the park at the many mothers enjoying their own lunches and activities with their families, and my thoughts began to drift to an alternative Mother's Day… one where I hadn't survived my illness on ECMO, where my two young sons had to face this usual day of celebration without their mum. Tears quietly pricked at my eyes and, in what would be the first time of many similar moments, I found myself wrestling with simultaneously contrasting emotions – joy and intense gratitude at being there, alive and whole, with my precious family, while at the very same time mourning a situation that so easily could have been very different to now. In that setting of warm autumn beauty on Mother's Day it was confusing and upsetting, and would be the start of many experiences of survivor's panic that would wash over me in the coming months.

After lunch and present opening of my mum's Mother's Day gift, she then handed me a wrapped package of her own. Surprised, I opened it to find a beautifully presented journal, filled with her heartfelt daily entries from my time in hospital. It also contained the names of worship songs she'd listened to while I was in the coma, as well as bible verses and messages of prayer and encouragement that many people had sent to her and my dad during that time. I instinctively started reading it then and there, but as my eyes filled with tears I quickly realised I would need time and solitude to slowly absorb the information, scenarios and emotions that spilled from the pages, just as I had with Matt's journal. When I did read it over the following days, I was incredibly moved by the way in which my mum's words offered a deeply personal perspective on the same events during my week in the coma – combined with Matt's journal, as well as the one my nurses had kept, they provided me with a precious gift of understanding from that time that I'd have never otherwise known.

We ended that special Sunday with a family photo, the four of us sitting on a log under a towering golden-leafed tree, arms relaxed around each other. Such a normal, natural thing to do on Mother's Day, yet the significance of that moment – of physically being there to take the photo, whole and *alive* – was so very strong. We are filled with togetherness, and each of us wears a smile. Soft smiles that reflect the beauty of the day but also hint at the effects of the trauma our family has gone through - battle-weary, still bruised. It will take time to heal. A lot of time. But we'll do it together. A framed copy of that photo sits in our living room and I still look at it every day – a precious reminder of God's goodness and provision.

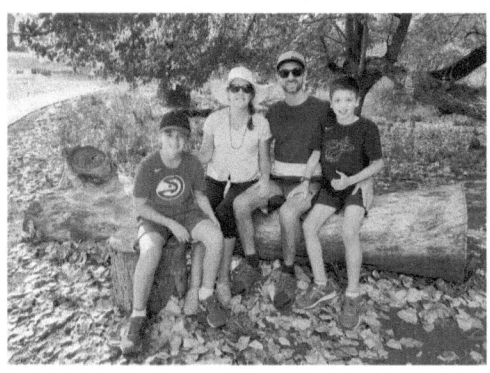

Chapter Twenty Two

It didn't take long after coming home from hospital to begin to realise how widely known what had happened to me in that first week in April was. Early conversations with Matt and my parents had revealed the practical and emotional support so many people locally had shown to our family, as well as the amazing extent to which people across the country – many unknown to us – had been praying for my survival and recovery. The heartfelt text messages, phone calls, emails, cards and flower deliveries that started pouring in after my return home so beautifully showed that. I felt humbled and grateful beyond words.

What did prove to become an emotional challenge, however, was the dawning realisation that literally thousands of people knew what had happened to me – or at least a version of events – before I even understood the situation myself. As mentioned earlier, the time during which I was hospitilised was one of heightened emotions – fear, confusion, exhaustion and uncertainty were all being experienced in communities across Australia, including ours. Government mandates dictated who could and couldn't enter workplaces, restaurants, entertainment venues and recreation centres, newspapers filled multiple pages with highly emotive covid-related stories, and the nightly news led with daily case numbers in WA, highlighting those hospitalised and in intensive care. One evening in the ICU my nurse had turned the TV on in time for the 6pm bulletin, and I cannot adequately describe what an intensely strange and unsettling experience it was to lie in my hospital bed and see those figures displayed prominently on the screen, my deeply traumatic experience so publicly represented as a statistic on state-wide news.

The sense of fear and uncertainty felt in the community meant that my critical illness and time spent on life support became a topic of shocked horror for so many. I was a fit forty-one year old, an active mother of two young boys who loved being in the outdoors. People were confused and scared – really scared, I would later find out in a number of conversations – by the extreme outcome of my illness. They questioned whether it could happen to them, their partner, their daughter. By this stage, covid infection was becoming widespread across WA, with a large proportion of the wider community having contracted it. And yet no one knew anyone else to have responded in the way I did. Stories were shared, information passed on, understandings and conclusions made. My deeply personal, traumatic experience – which I was far from comprehending myself – was, for better or for worse, very much the topic of public discussion.

This became very apparent one evening a couple of weeks after returning home from hospital, when two former work colleagues of mine kindly delivered a meal to our home. The couple had been part of the prayer group who happened to be meeting the evening I was flown to Perth and put on life support, the eight of them experiencing the tangible presence of a spiritual battle that filled the room as they pushed back against death in intercessory prayer. One of the couple had taken on work fitting curtain railings, and he now shared with us how he'd been chatting with a client in her home during a recent job, and talk had turned towards the amount of covid cases in the community. When the lady commented that most people seemed to be recovering from the virus well, she then added, "Except for that woman I've heard about who's on life support in a coma after getting covid. I think she's not expected to survive. Apparently she's a mum of young children too. It's very sad". My friend quickly realised that his client was talking about me, and told her that we'd used to work together. When it became apparent this lady didn't know me personally, my friend shared more about my situation, including the amazing amount of prayer interceding for my full recovery. It was for this reason he was now enthusiastically relaying the conversation to Matt and me. From my traumatised perspective though, the events of those two weeks were still incredibly raw and deeply confusing, and so when our friends left a short time later I sat at our dining table and truly sobbed. It was the most I'd cried since coming home from hospital. I cried for the conversations that were held about whether I'd live or die while I lay in a coma, unaware that my life even hung in the balance. I cried for the knowledge that so many people – especially strangers – had had during that week, while I still lacked so much understanding even now. I cried for the children of families who'd known more about the dire situation of my illness than my own boys had understood at the time – indeed, when our sons returned to school two weeks after I'd come home from hospital, they were met with many well-meaning and loving, but nonetheless confronting, admissions from schoolmates such as "We prayed for your mum when she was in hospital because she might have died". I cried for what I now felt acutely as being the local 'poster girl' for covid infection gone spectacularly wrong – known by name in the conversations of strangers, talked about by so many in the community.

I sobbed in my confusion. I knew that having thousands of people know of my illness had led to so many bold and heartfelt prayers for my survival and full recovery. I praised God for that every day. But being so early in my post-coma recovery, the overwhelm that I felt by having my traumatic experience so publicly known – and completely out of my control – was acute.

And so began a journey of surrender, in a way I'd never experienced before, that God would lead me on over the coming months.

I continued to travel to and from Perth for scans, tests and medical checks over the following months and, in between, I relished all of the 'firsts' since coming home from hospital as we slowly returned to some semblance of normality in our family routine.

Our first family walk along the estuary as the sun set in a spectacular golden glow – holding hands with Matt as our boys rode on their scooters ahead, it was a walk that was gentle and fairly short in duration before I became fatigued, but an incredible reminder of how far I'd come less than two months after being in the coma.

Our family's return to our church, greeted by the same sea of smiling faces that had appeared in the video sent to me in intensive care. I'd seen or spoken with many of these people over the past two months, during the visits, meal deliveries and phone calls that had lovingly poured in, but to be back in our building of worship with the voices of our faith family joining together in praise was an overwhelmingly emotional moment.

The first Saturday I returned to our boys' footy matches on a chilly but clear morning – overcome with gratitude of being able to take part in watching my children's weekend sport, an activity I'd admittedly often taken for granted in the past.

And then, when I finally started driving again, the first day of returning to the school run, collecting my boys in the afternoon and delighting in watching them walk towards the car, bags casually slung on their shoulders, chatting animatedly with each other – a simple, everyday image I vowed not to forget.

Another 'first' was the day I returned to the seemingly straightforward task of buying our family's weekly fresh produce at our local farmers' market, about two months after my illness. Since I'd been in hospital Matt or my parents had taken on the task of food shopping, allowing for my recovery and protecting my immuno-compromised body from infections in those early weeks. On this day, I decided the task of picking through apples and pondering over meats would prove a solid step forward in returning to normality, although my apprehensive nerves as I drove to the shops betrayed how I was really feeling. The local farmers' market is a very popular place, and bumping into one familiar person after another while shopping is the norm. It would be my first excursion outside of hospital to a busy, people-filled space, and I wasn't sure what to expect after spending the past two months in a gentle bubble of recovery. Sure enough, it was a market visit that was well and truly out of the ordinary, with many people I knew reacting with open joy and tears upon seeing me for the first time post-coma. I was incredibly moved by their display of emotion but, as we stood there talking, I struggled massively to articulate to so many people the enormity of what I'd been through, and I found that sharing about what had happened while standing in such a public, busy space soon left me feeling emotionally overwhelmed. And then there was the starkly different response of others – the small handful of acquaintances who saw me but clearly didn't know what to say, their uncertainty written all over their faces. They would stare at me, then duck their heads to avoid making eye contact and, although it felt confusing to me, I also strangely understood. For some, it would be hard to know where to start in conversation with someone who's so recently faced death, been in a coma, put on life support – especially if it's the first time of contact since the event. It takes courage for a person to put aside their own feelings of discomfort and uncertainty and reach out to someone who's experienced suffering – often, a simple "I'm so sorry for what you've been through. It's really good to see you now" goes a long way in acknowledging pain and reducing the loneliness of trauma. Many years earlier I'd experienced a similar situation after suffering a pregnancy loss. I'd returned to work and a colleague, clearly overcome by not knowing what to say upon first seeing me, did a very quick U-turn in the office hallway and wordlessly retreated in the opposite direction. With no judgement whatsoever, I learnt a very important lesson that day which I've continued to live by – to never let my own feelings of discomfort or self-consciousness stop me from reaching out to somebody who's hurting. If they don't want to talk about their circumstances further that's OK, and very much their choice, but I firmly believe most people will feel loved by simply having their pain acknowledged. Now, in the months after my experience in hospital, I appreciated all the more the many precious people who did exactly that.

Chapter Twenty Three

Imagine being in a car accident, sustaining such critical injuries that you're placed in a coma on life support. You wake six days later with no memory of the accident itself, but through the explanations of others over the following days you begin to understand a little of what happened. While you're in ICU the TV news offers daily data on serious road accidents, as well as statistics on the likelihood of being involved in one. When you come home from hospital, newspapers are filling their pages with stories about the ongoing threat of driving, and everybody in the community is talking about car crashes – who's been involved in one, the extent of their injuries, where it happened, the danger of driving a car, the chances of it happening again. Everybody has a road accident story to share – but then none of them reflect the extreme circumstances of yours. If it feels like a desperately poor analogy, it's probably because it is. But it can be very hard to articulate exactly how difficult it was to mentally and emotionally heal from a traumatic experience that was caused by an event the entire community – the entire nation, in fact – seemed fixated on. I couldn't escape the daily discussions, analyses and opinions on covid infections, and that forced me to think about it constantly. 'Stay safe out there' became something of a public motto, and yet the saturated attention on the virus led me to feel anything but safe. In the weeks and months after leaving hospital, the uncertainty and fear that was constantly reinforced in media coverage, public announcements and even everyday conversations meant I constantly felt a confusing and uncontrollable sense of life-threatening danger. It lurked in every interaction with visitors, every hug, every public outing. Our boys' school continued to release regular updates on the number of students currently infected with covid, meaning even my children's place of education became a threat in my mind. Combined with a lack of concrete answers as to why my body had responded so severely to the virus – and whether that reaction would happen again – the seeds of anxiety and panic embedded themselves in my thoughts and began to steadily grow.

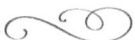

I also felt an aching loneliness at times that stemmed from the isolating uniqueness of my experience and not knowing anyone else who shared that understanding. The sickest patient in intensive care... a covid-related ICU statistic on the TV news... extreme immune response to spike protein... the most severe case in Western Australia... the only person in WA to be placed on ECMO life support for covid-related cardiogenic shock... descriptives that were quite sensational for most people who'd heard of my situation, but brought about a deep sense of confusion and 'otherness' for me. I longed for some kind of communal support group that could connect me with others who'd experienced being on ECMO life support, who understood the trauma of waking from a coma with no idea of where they were or how they'd gotten there. I battled against frequent feelings of dislocation, finding it difficult to reconnect with everyday life and community. This was especially so when the final remaining covid restrictions were lifted just a month after I returned home from hospital, and the eagerness of most people to throw off the extreme heaviness of the past two years and embrace a 'normal' life again felt jarringly apparent. On the one hand, I completely understood – if I hadn't gone through what I did, I would have felt exactly the same way. But the reality of my experience, and its profound impact on me, meant I couldn't share in that response anymore, and I grieved that.

It was some months after coming out of hospital, while reading the book *I'm Not Crazy, I'm Just A Little Unwell* by Australian journalist Leigh Hatcher [2] in which he describes his years-long journey through chronic fatigue syndrome, that I found understanding of how I was feeling. In his own publication, Leigh discusses another book called *Surviving Survival*, which was written by four doctors in Sydney who'd explored the unique challenges faced by survivors of serious illness to reconnect back into a sense of normal life. As part of their findings, which Leigh wrote about in his book, the authors concluded that,

[A survivor's] sense of identity had been disrupted. It is difficult to exist as a survivor, because their views and values have changed, while people around them have not. Their experiences have been such that they have been made incorrigibly aware of the limitations and frailties of the human body. The illness had changed the person they were before the illness.[3]

These words resonated so deeply with me, and I felt a surprisingly emotional sense of relief at the understanding. My experience of critical illness in the hospital, and everything that had happened during that time of isolation, was still so raw, confusing and *abnormal*, and that place of contrast meant I now often felt a sense of existing on the periphery of everyday life and community. Personally confronting my mortality had also brought into sharp focus the frailty of life. If we're honest, most of us will picture our final days on this earth to be in old age, after a life well lived and with a lead-up well prepared. When we're under a certain age, we talk freely and lightly about which songs we'd like played at our funeral, or joke about what we expect people to say in our eulogy. Facing up to my mortality as a forty-one year old wife and mother of two young boys in such a real and abrupt way had impacted me greatly. My strong faith in the promise of God's Word meant I'd always held a confident assurance of eternal life after earthly death, and that certainly hadn't changed. Now more than ever, God's purpose for my life as part of His creation – to glorify Him, be in personal relationship with Him and find deep joy in Him, as well as being in loving fellowship with others – became my absolute anchor when everything else lacked certainty and felt uncontrollably unsettled.

It was therefore hugely encouraging to read in Leigh Hatcher's book one of the conclusions the authors of *Surviving Survival* had arrived at when exploring the sense of life dislocation many survivors experienced:

The first and most common way of handling all this seems to be the use of 'anchor points', strong values and beliefs that stand their stead in turbulence.[3]

For me, choosing to place my trust in God's unfailing love and steadfast promises in the face of so much uncertainty was my 'anchor for the soul' (Hebrews 6:19).

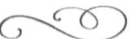

And so it was on a rainy mid-winter morning that I arrived at a place of surrender.

To describe the three months after coming home from hospital as an emotional rollercoaster couldn't be a more accurate cliché. My indescribable gratitude at being fully healed and alive intermingled with an acute sense of survivor's guilt if I felt anything other than pure joy. I was intensely thankful that I had both of my legs intact, but my thoughts were often shocked by the what ifs of an alternative scenario. I craved talking to people about my time in hospital, in an attempt to make sense of what had happened, but struggled to fully communicate the trauma of the experience. My confused thoughts questioned over and over how the situation could have gone downhill so quickly and intensely – a coma, my family not given the chance to say goodbye, life support (*life support!*... how??) – all the while praising God for His unfailing presence and protection during that time. There was still so much I couldn't remember, and I constantly searched to know more to fill in the blanks – but when some of those missing puzzle pieces did arrive, the sudden memory of a particular moment before or during my time in hospital triggered an avalanche of physical and emotional panic. Filled with overwhelming gratitude at being alive and present, I was now conscious of living fully in every moment – and yet I often felt tied to dark thoughts of an alternative reality, where a grieving Matt was without his wife, and our young boys without their mum. Having children forced me to stay engaged with life – when the temptation to isolate in fear of further illness threatened to take hold, my desire to be involved in our boys' activities, cheer at their sporting matches, attend their school assemblies and be a part of church together as a whole family meant I had to step out in faith, day after day.

While the specialists admitted they couldn't tell me if I'd experience a similar reaction if and when I contracted covid a second time, they agreed that the severity of my immune system's initial response meant the extremely high level of antibodies produced would give me a solid level of protection in any future cases. While I did take reassurance in that, my long-held confidence in a strong and healthy immune system to do its protective job in my body had been shattered, and I felt deeply confused and disoriented by that. The trauma of ending up in a coma was also still very raw, and so the admission that whether history would repeat itself next time was unknown constantly hung over me. But when that uncertainty threatened to distress me to the point of debilitating panic, Matt encouraged me to take strength in Jesus' promise of an abundant life:

The thief comes only to steal and kill and destroy; I have come that they may have life, and have it to the full. (John 10:10)

I knew deep in my soul that I hadn't survived my illness to then live a life of isolating fear and solitude, and yet I couldn't reconcile how to 'stay safe' and not end up back on life support when the threat still appeared to loom. I experienced regular moments of guilt that I even felt such anxiety – I'd been fully healed after all! Shouldn't I be living in a constant state of joy and thankfulness?

Like I said, emotional rollercoaster.

It was on that morning in mid-July, three months after coming home from hospital, that the fear felt overwhelming. Matt was at work, and our boys were spending a day of their school holidays with their cousin. On my knees in the loungeroom, weeping with the crushing burden of anxiety, I knew without question I needed to truly hand over my fears to God and leave them at His feet. I couldn't keep trying to do this battle on my own – nor was I ever supposed to.

I've never been a journaller, despite my training and career as a journalist. But on that day, almost instinctively, I found a notebook and began writing, pouring out my fears one after the other in words on the page.

Fear of having died without being able to prepare for it or say goodbye.
Fear of my boys being without a mother, and Matt losing his wife.
Fear of being trapped.
Fear of ending up in a coma again without knowing it.
Fear that my body is weak, and will succumb to the virus again.
Fear of people not understanding what happened to me, and making their own judgements.
Fear of illness, and people carrying viruses.
Fear of loneliness.

As I wrote, something incredible happened – God clearly revealed to me what I needed to *surrender* to Him first in order to truly release my fears.

My life – literally whether I live or die.
Certainty.
Control.
My children.

My reputation.
The truth.

As I began writing this new list, I spoke the words out loud as I visualised physically laying each of these areas of surrender at the foot of the Cross. What happened next astounded me. With every spoken surrender, I felt a physical lifting of weight from my shoulders – a literal release of the burden that I was experiencing, tangibly in that very moment. Months of anxiety, fear and confusion fell away as I knelt on the floor, surrendering complete control over the things most important to me to the One who was in control all along.

The sense of freedom was profound.

God is our refuge and strength... Therefore we will not fear, though the earth give way. (Psalm 46:1...2) – written in my journal that day.

Moving forward from that day, it's an ongoing prayer that sees me returning to God over and again to keep handing my fears to Him when they arise – because they still do, even now. I've discovered this surrender does not equate to weakness, but instead an immense strength and peace in wholly trusting in God's sovereignty over my life.

In His strength, I refuse to accept a life bound by fear, worry and anxiety.

Even though I walk through the valley of the shadow of death I will fear no evil, for you are with me... your goodness and unfailing love will follow me all the days of my life. (Psalm 23: 4...6)

Chapter Twenty Four

It was always going to be an emotional moment. How much so, though, Matt and I were completely unprepared for. Time had now marched into the summer heat of early January, nine months since I'd been in the coma, and I'd travelled to Perth for an ultrasound, ECG and echocardiogram at Fiona Stanley Hospital. Weeks before my appointment, Matt and I had begun talking about the idea of meeting with Dr Chris Allen, the ICU Intensivist who'd led the team caring for me so skillfully while I was on ECMO life support. I'd been in contact with Dr Allen a number of times via phone and email in the months after leaving hospital – I'd even sent photos to him in celebration of physical achievements and special family moments, which he'd always replied to with encouragement. But I hadn't seen Dr Allen face to face since being in ICU, and Matt had never met him in person, given he wasn't allowed to enter the hospital during my time there. Having never had any experience of intensive care before my illness, we had no idea of the protocols. Was it the done thing to contact an ICU Intensivist to say you'd really like to meet with them? Would he be too busy saving lives to even have the time for that? With a little nervousness I sent Dr Allen an email, telling him about my appointment at the hospital and asking whether it would be possible to meet afterwards, and was thrilled when he replied saying he would try his hardest to make it work. And so Matt and I headed to Perth early on that Monday morning in January, with the plan to call Dr Allen from the hospital's Advanced Heart Failure Clinic after my scans and appointment were finished. We had no expectations of the time to come – if all we could have was a short ten minutes with Dr Allen to express our deep gratitude in person we'd be hugely thankful for that. It was late morning when I called his number, and Dr Allen told us to wait outside the entrance to the hospital as he'd come straight down from ICU. In our nervousness, Matt and I joked about how the situation felt like a blind date – considering I'd never seen Dr Allen without PPE, and Matt hadn't met him at all, we weren't even sure who we were looking for every time the hospital's automatic doors opened. But when Dr Allen arrived he walked straight towards us, and I was very relieved to see the face of a smiling, friendly-looking doctor, and not the orange-beaked duck that I remembered from my confused time in ICU.

It was hard to know what to say at first. After all, how do you find adequate words to express your gratitude to the man who helped to save your life, or that of your wife's? But Dr Allen led the way in conversation, saying how wonderful it was to both see me again looking so healthy and well, and to finally be able to meet Matt in person. After about five minutes of talking, when Dr Allen asked if we now wanted to visit the intensive care unit with him, Matt and I looked at each other in surprise, agreeing with nervous anticipation that it was something we'd very much like.

Right from the start, Dr Allen clearly recognised the importance of the visit. With Matt having not been allowed to be at the hospital during my time there, and my memories either non-existent or skewed by trauma, confusion and post-coma medication, Dr Allen talked us through every relevant part of the hospital as we walked to ICU – where the ambulance transporting me from the airport would have arrived; the emergency doors through which I'd been wheeled; the room I'd been initially assessed in; the lift that had carried my bed and life-support equipment up and down multiple times for surgery, both before and during the coma; the operating theatre itself. Again, I experienced those conflicting emotions – desperate to know more to fill in the many distressing gaps, while at the same time feeling a sense of disconnect from what I was seeing, as though it had happened to someone else. And then we passed through the large double doors into the intensive care unit, and I felt my heart begin to hammer in my chest. Matt's hand had been holding mine the whole time, and now I felt his grip gently tighten as I began to quietly shake all over – I suddenly remembered being pushed down this very corridor in my bed on the way to the cardiology ward. As we walked past room after room towards Pod 4, one thought kept gnawing away at my mind, and then it hit me – everything seemed so *normal*, exactly like a busy ICU should look. It felt light and bright, with colorful posters and signs lining the walls. While many of the doctors and nurses walking past us wore surgical masks, there definitely wasn't a PPE gown or visor in sight. Doors leading into patient rooms were almost always open and, as we walked past, I discretely looked in to see visitors sitting by bedsides, holding the hands of their loved one or simply sitting quietly in a chair. Emotion washed over me and my eyes filled with tears as I registered the normalcy of visitors simply *being there*, their presence no doubt of huge comfort to their unwell loved one. I glanced at Matt and could see by the expression on his face that he was clearly overcome by similar thoughts to my own. As we continued to follow behind Dr Allen my heart started to pound even faster, and straight away I realised why – there, directly opposite a busy central doctors' and nurses' station, was my room. The space that had enclosed me for eleven days, shut off to the outside world and even the rest of the hospital. Despite the many gaps in my memory, I could very clearly picture being wheeled out of that doorway and into the corridor on my way to the cardiology unit. Sure enough, we stopped just outside the open entrance to the room, and Dr Allen confirmed my memory when he turned to Matt and said with obvious sensitivity, "And this is the room where Abbey was on ECMO". It was such a surreal moment – to be back in that very space, and now with Matt. I waited for the associated feelings of anxiety and fear to come over me... and yet they didn't. The atmosphere was so different from that of the one in my mind and memories. There were no boys frantically running past the door in the corridor trying to escape being caught. The medical staff milling at the desk opposite my room *looked* like doctors and nurses, not aliens in space suits. The oppressive sensations of darkness, heaviness and isolation were gone, replaced by bright lights, chattering voices and space to move. Again, I felt conflicting emotion – intense confusion by the reality I was seeing compared to my previous experience, coupled with overwhelming relief that it *was* so different. I found myself saying "This is *nothing* like it was when I was in here" to Matt over and over, as if to emphasise my deep need for that to be understood. For my husband, however, the emotion of finally being able to stand at the room in which I'd lain for almost a week, unresponsive in the depth of a coma, revealed itself and he began to weep quietly. The cruel burden he'd carried during that time – separated from his critically ill wife, unable to be by her side, holding her hand, protecting her – was both remembered and released by the presence of finally *being there*. I don't think Matt had been prepared for the intensity of the moment, and so he took some time to walk down the corridor, calming himself before he returned to Dr Allen and me. Just seconds later, a nurse walked out of the room we were standing in front of, and Dr Allen called her over to us, telling Matt and me "This is someone you'll want to meet". Turning to the nurse, Dr Allen said, "Kristie, this is Abbey Spinelli and her husband Matt. Abbey was on ECMO in Pod Four in April last year". The response was instant – Kristie startled, her eyes suddenly pricking with tears, and I turned quickly to see Matt's face also flooded with emotion. Sensing my confusion, he explained "I spoke with Kristie on the phone many times while you were in the coma. She was the nurse who took the video call that first allowed me to see you, and to see the life support machine and your room." Matt turned to Kristie, his eyes now filled with tears. "I was so thankful for those calls, and also for the way you cared for Abbey in the coma. I remember you even washed and plaited her hair, which you proudly showed me over one of the video calls." I was overcome by emotion at what I was hearing, picturing the distressing scenario in which these conversations would have been held. And in that moment I suddenly realised how important our meeting today would be to Matt's healing as well as my own.

In the conversation that followed, Kristie emphasised a number of times, "It's just so wonderful to see you coming back to intensive care to visit us, walking and upright!". At this point, Matt and I didn't realise the significance of her words, but later we would come to understand the emotional impact that my healthy return to the ICU had on, not just us, but the ECMO medical team as well. Kristie was soon called away to the needs of a patient, and Dr Allen continued to introduce Matt and me to a number of doctors and nurses who'd been working in the intensive care unit at the time of my hospitalisation. We were amazed to find that all Dr Allen had to say were those same words – "This is Abbey Spinelli. She was on ECMO in Pod Four in April last year" – and everyone we met knew straight away who I was, their faces lighting up in recognition. Over and over, I was told how incredibly well I was looking, what a joy it was to see me upright and walking through ICU, how thankful the medical staff were that I'd come back to visit – even though it was us desperately wanting to thank *them*! It was deeply humbling and incredibly emotional.

By now we'd been with Dr Allen for over an hour. Matt and I were both very aware of respecting his time restraints, unsure of in what capacity he was working at the hospital that day. There was, however, a lot more we longed to talk about with Dr Allen, and so Matt said rather hesitantly, "We'd love to buy you a coffee in the hospital café and spend some more time talking with you, if that's possible? Although we fully understand if you can't". It was then we learnt that Dr Allen wasn't officially rostered on at the hospital that day, and had instead come in specifically to meet with us. We were very touched, and it made us deeply appreciate the time spent with him even more.

We settled with our drinks at a table outside the café downstairs, and began what would end up being an almost two hour conversation with Dr Allen. Still trying to make sense of so much that had happened, we asked question after question to the doctor whose care for me while on ECMO had helped to save my life. How and when was it first decided that ECMO life support was my only chance of survival? Was Dr Allen involved with the communication between the two hospitals that led to me being flown to Perth? This is when we discovered yet another way in which God had held His protective hand over the situation – the young doctor rostered on at Bunbury Hospital that first day of April had not long transferred from Fiona Stanley Hospital, where she'd completed part of her training under Dr Allen and developed an understanding of ECMO life support. In her wisdom – and therefore more quickly than might otherwise have been – it was determined that my severe illness was not respiratory in cause (as was often previously the case with covid-related complications, particularly in the northern hemisphere), but heart related. When my condition continued to deteriorate, and cardiogenic shock was diagnosed, this young doctor's recent knowledge of ECMO, and her connection with Dr Allen, played an important part in the decision to fly me to Perth to access the high-risk but life-saving machine.

As our conversation with Dr Allen deepened, our questions kept on coming. Given I was the most critically unwell patient in ICU at the time, did the doctors expect me to survive, even on ECMO? Was there a time limit as to how long they would have left me on the life support machine? And the question, asked by Matt, that I'll never forget, so emotional was it to hear – "If Abbey had been about to pass away, would I have been allowed into her room to say goodbye?" Nine months later, it was a question that still clearly carried the trauma of the restrictive circumstances at the time.

We talked openly with Dr Allen about the huge difficulty of being separated during my time in hospital, and the significant impact the isolation restrictions had had on my initial distress. We shared honestly about the challenges of healing afterwards in an environment of fear, uncertainty and misunderstanding, as well as the heightened community interest in what had happened to me. We described the prayer chain that had spread across the country and to other parts of the world, covering me as I lay in the coma, Matt and my family as they lived through that week at home, and the medical team as they skillfully cared for me. And then Dr Allen shared with us the challenges and emotions of working in a medical specialty – intensive care and, more specifically, ECMO – that comes with a much higher incidence of mortality and life-impacting outcomes than other areas of care in a hospital. He confirmed that the survival rate of patients on ECMO is less than fifty percent, and for those who do survive, half again will be impacted by chronic health issues requiring long-term support and treatment. When confronted with ECMO statistics through the words of a skilled specialist whose work is immersed in the reality of this level of life support, I was yet again overwhelmed by the understanding of my full and complete healing. Dr Allen's honesty about the challenges involved in caring for such critically ill patients gave us greater understanding, and it was then we realised why so many of the staff we'd met with earlier had expressed their emotion and gratitude at seeing me return to the ICU looking so healthy and strong – in their field of work, particularly when it came to ECMO, that was never a given. While Matt and I were so very thankful for our time spent at the hospital that morning, we now understood that our return to visit there meant more than we'd realised to the medical staff as well.

Acknowledging how incredibly gracious and generous Dr Allen had been in giving us almost three hours of his time, we ended our meeting together with a hug – filled with the intense gratitude that Matt and I had struggled to put into adequate words. And then, with lifted hearts and the recognition that something very special had happened that morning, we headed home.

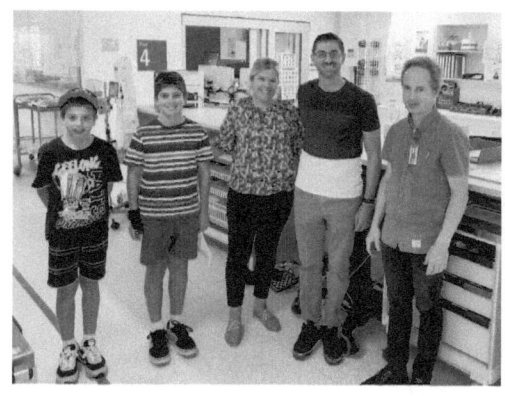

Visiting Dr Chris Allen in Pod Four, this time with Coby and Jesaia

Chapter Twenty Five

The flashback, when it came, was as physical as it was sudden. It was an evening in mid-January, just two weeks after our emotional visit to the ICU, and I was standing at the kitchen sink washing dishes while worship music played softly in the background. Deep in thought, I didn't notice as one song melted into the next, and a distinctively deep, gravelly voice filled the room. Without warning I was overwhelmed by a visceral reaction like none I'd ever experienced, its immediacy and intensity leaving me literally breathless. Within seconds – uncontrollably, and before I'd even consciously registered the start of the song – my heart began racing, sweat and a prickly heat flushed over my face, my whole body started shaking and I felt dizzy and lightheaded. Despite standing freely, I was overcome by the sensation of being pinned down, restricted in both movement and understanding. An oppressive heaviness flooded over me and, seemingly without control, my mind was instantly transported back to the images of the coma. The Akubra-clad elderly man, his head tilted down, sitting on the verandah of his homestead. The laughing, friendly faces of a group of women, all with brightly bleached hair and lipstick-red mouths. The lion face with its thick, wild mane. The swirling, dizzying kaleidoscope of colours. I leant against the kitchen sink, steadying myself as my whole body shook and my heart raced. Despite my confusion and shock over the intensity of the sudden flashback, I knew without doubt that I'd heard that song, 'I Surrender' – and specifically, the distinct, gravelly voice singing the lyrics – while I was in the coma. When Matt came into the kitchen a few minutes later he found me quietly crying, as equally shaken up by the physicality of the experience as I was overcome by emotion that I now had another memory link to that otherwise dark void in time. It wasn't my first flashback since coming home from hospital – I'd had a handful of those already as some of the puzzle pieces dropped back into my memory – but it was by far the most physically and emotionally impacting.

Another one would hit me with full force a few weeks later, as I walked along a bush track near our home. Listening to music through my earphones, I hadn't registered the jogger who was running closer behind me until he was nearly ready to pass. The distinct pounding sound of running footsteps that suddenly invaded my music instantly took me back to my ICU room and the distress at hearing what I thought were boys being chased in the corridor outside. In my thoughts I was instantly no longer on the bush track near my home, but instead trapped to an ever-moving bed, begging my nurse to help the boys to safety. My heart hammering, I instinctively turned on the track and screamed loudly at the realisation that someone was right behind me. The young male jogger, who now stopped short, looked understandably shocked and began stumbling over a repeated apology. Shaking all over from both memories and mortification I, in turn, began apologising profusely to *him*, upset by my seemingly uncontrollable reaction to the sensation I'd experienced. As the young man hesitantly jogged away, and I began praying that he would understand he'd done nothing wrong to warrant his apologies to me, I knew I needed help.

A few weeks after leaving hospital, I'd been discussing the necessity of seeing a professional counsellor with Dr Allen, who'd phoned me to follow up on my ongoing recovery. He shared with me that around half of patients surviving critical illness in hospital will go on to experience post-intensive care syndrome (PICS), of which the physical, mental and emotional symptoms can present or last from a few months to a number of years. Add to the mix that I'd woken from a coma with no understanding of where I was or how I'd gotten there, during one of the most restrictive and disorienting times our world had seen in recent history, and there was a strong likelihood I'd benefit from professional help in working through all that had happened. However Dr Allen encouraged me not to put pressure on myself as to the 'right' time to seek counselling, saying if I did feel the need to speak to someone in this way, "it could be over the coming months, or it might even be after a year or more has passed." I very much appreciated Dr Allen's wisdom on this, and the sense of freedom it gave me to avoid placing expectations on the healing process.

Now, around nine months after our phone conversation, I knew I needed professional support. The many black holes in my understanding of that critical time in hospital still confused and upset me, and I felt overwhelmed and confronted by the memories that did return, with their tendency to crash into my brain without warning. I also realised my need to regularly talk about what had happened, as well as my ongoing recovery, as a way to try to make sense of the emotions and thoughts that often tumbled through my mind. Matt and my parents were always available as a listening ear and a willing source of understanding and comfort, but I recognised the importance of speaking with someone who was objective to the trauma we'd all experienced in different ways.

Over the following months, through my time with the counsellor, I began to understand exactly how hard the brain must work to link together and process memories that have been deeply fractured. My fragmented recall of events, from before, during and after the coma, stemmed from a mixture of critical illness, medicinal impact and the emotional trauma of the circumstances. I accepted that I might never remember much more than I already did from my time spent in darkness during the coma, but it upset me greatly that I could barely recall any memory of the forty-eight hours leading up to being put on ECMO life support, despite being awake for most of that time. And so when I began to experience a strong emotional response – heart hammering, hands shaking, head dizzying – every time an ambulance would pass me on the road, its siren blaring and lights flashing, I felt confused and frustrated. From the information I'd been told, I knew I *had* travelled from hospital to airport, and then airport to hospital, in an ambulance under emergency conditions. And I had experienced a very short, sharp memory of waking in the ambulance on the way to Fiona Stanley Hospital, before succumbing once again to an unknown darkness. But surely this wasn't enough to warrant the reaction my mind and body now seemed to automatically respond with when faced with a passing ambulance? And so I learnt about the difference between data memory –

that associated with fact-based information, and often more challenging to recall – and the highly-engaging reaction of emotional memory. In those experiences of heightened emotional response, the counsellor encouraged me to re-train my thoughts on the help the patient in the ambulance was receiving, the expertise of the paramedics, and the care of the medical professionals involved in that moment – thereby creating a new association through melding the memory.

And then summer drifted slowly into autumn, and to mark the double-digits milestone of our youngest son Coby turning ten a few months earlier, my dad organised a special Pop-Grandson scenic flight through the local aero club. It was a perfect day for flying – a cool air with not a hint of wind, and clear blue skies. Following the flight the small plane landed smoothly, and the two passengers joined Matt, Jesaia and me by the gate overlooking the tarmac, full of stories of what they'd seen during the hour-long loop down the coast. As they talked, an ambulance drove past us on the way to a nearby hangar, where a Royal Flying Doctor Service plane sat waiting. I hadn't noticed the plane earlier, and so I now walked a little closer to the gate, watching discretely as the back doors of the ambulance were opened and a patient was wheeled out. Without warning tears began filling my eyes as I took in the scene – the ambulance, the plane, the hospital gurney, the medical and flight workers. All missing pieces of a larger puzzle that made up a memoryless week. A crucial part of that early-April Saturday I was flown to Perth, critically ill and fighting for life – a day of which I'd had many a conversation about, but still felt as though belonged to someone else. And so now I cried in gratitude, thankful for the gift of visual confirmation I was being given today – I *had* travelled to the airport in an ambulance like the one now sitting before me; I *had* been wheeled across that tarmac on a gurney just like the one I could see; I *had* been cared for by medical attendants like those there today; I *had* been carefully loaded into an RFDS plane, maybe even that very same one. The scene that was unfolding today didn't involve me, but it painted a much-needed picture in my mind of what it *would have* been like on that day. It brought realness to a situation that I previously couldn't grasp through lack of memory and understanding. And I was thankful for the gentleness of the moment. The scene before me didn't appear frantic or stressed, and this puzzle piece didn't come with the shock of a sudden memory or flashback. It felt helpful and healing, rather than abrasive and distressing.

In that moment I prayed for the patient and medical workers inside the plane now taxiing down the runway. And then, along with my family, it was time to go home.

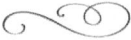

Months later, I lay in bed late at night waiting for sleep to come. Without warning, and despite not having been thinking about anything related to my illness that evening, I suddenly began hearing in my mind the distinct beeping sounds of hospital machinery. Instantly I was transported back to being in my ICU bed, overcome by the sensation of being unable to move freely. I even began to smell the sharp hospital odour of chemical disinfectant, which before now I hadn't experienced. With my eyes closed, my senses seemed to be working together in a powerful bid to convince me that I was no longer lying in my bed at home, healthy and well, but instead back in the isolation of Pod Four in the intensive care unit. As incredibly unnerving as the experience was though, on this particular night my automatic reaction wasn't to enter into panic or anxiety. Rather, with a sense of almost curiosity I allowed myself to acknowledge each distinct sensation, intrigued by the intensity of it rather than fearing it. Recognising how strong and clear this sudden sensory memory was, I reminded myself out loud that it was exactly that – a memory, of a place and time different to now – and that it was nothing to fear.

Mind, body and soul, so intricate and holistic in its connection – the wonder of human Creation. I drifted into sleep a short time later, my spirit at peace.

Chapter Twenty Six

My heart may sing to you and not be silent (Psalm 30:12)

My exhausted and battered, yet healed heart had vowed on that final night in hospital to not stay silent in singing the praises of its Almighty Healer. And God provided many, many opportunities over the months after I came home from hospital to share with others – people I knew, and those I didn't whom I came to know – of His miraculous works and faithfulness. In October of that year, six months after the coma, Matt and I were invited to publicly share our testimony of God's healing at our church, Australind Baptist Church. We accepted, and so began an ongoing conversation with the one who heals.

"God, I can't do this. You know I have panic attacks when I speak publicly. I said yes, but I actually can't do this."

It came from a place of fear. Fourteen years earlier, while working as a breakfast newsreader at a Perth radio station, I'd experienced a very distressing and deeply humiliating panic attack live on air. It had followed the pregnancy loss of our first baby, and many weeks of going through the motions of publicly hiding the pain behind the scenes, putting on a strong, confident voice while reporting the daily news each hour. When the panic attack came mid-bulletin it was sudden, physical and very public. Gasping for air, literally unable to speak, I did the only thing I could think of to escape the suffocation – I ripped my headphones off and ran out of the news booth, leaving dead air on the radio. I had never suffered a panic attack before that day, and yet that one extreme moment – live on air – became the catalyst for years of intensely physical panic every time I had to speak publicly in front of more than one or two people.

And now I'd committed to speaking in front of almost two hundred people, sharing about the healing of a trauma that was still very much ongoing.

In the weeks leading up to that Sunday in October, the panic constantly bubbled just below the surface. My heart would race, my hands would shake, I'd feel an overwhelming need to vomit – and that was just *thinking* about getting up on the stage. And so my conversation with God became a daily one.

"God, I actually can't do this. Matt can speak, and I'll still sit next to him on the stage."

"God, I really can't do this. I can't speak well. My jaw tenses up. My muscles tighten. I shake all over. I can't breathe properly. How can I possibly share our testimony like this?"

But also, "Yes, God. I feel your conviction on this. I vowed in my hospital room not to be silent in speaking of your works. You're opening this door. May my words glorify your name. But please Lord, take away my panic."

And yet, "God, I'm still shaking. I feel terrified. Matt is feeling nervous, but I'm having full-blown anxiety. Please be the breath in my lungs to pour out your praise. But how can I share my testimony if I'm crying with panic?"

This continued until the morning of that day, when I sat on the stage with Matt in front of almost two hundred people and shared our testimony of the life-changing power of prayer and a miraculous healing.

But God was also healing me on that stage.

Hours before I'd been close to vomiting with physical panic at the thought of speaking so publicly... and yet now, after fourteen years, that grip was broken and released.

In nervous faith, we said yes to having our testimony – with my shaking voice and vulnerable honesty – placed on YouTube. Our deeply personal trauma, open to anyone to hear. Complete surrender. And God has used it in ways beyond our imagination, as only He can do. Countless connections and stories shared with people who've seen it, including those we didn't know before. So many opportunities to praise the name of our Almighty God.

Two weeks later I opened my bible to the book of Exodus, and began crying as I read the story of Moses, who was appointed by God to lead the enslaved Israelites out of Egypt. Filled with doubt and insecurity over his own capabilities, Moses expresses his lack of confidence to God, lamenting that he is not a strong speaker.

"O Lord, I have never been eloquent, neither in the past nor since you have spoken to your servant. I am slow of speech and tongue… please send someone else to do it." (Exodus 4:10…13)

I knew that panic intimately. The anxiety Moses expressed, over the thought of speaking publicly, felt as though it were my own.

Please Lord… use someone else to speak.

And yet God had replied to Moses,

"Who gave man his mouth?... Is it not I, the Lord? Now go; I will help you speak and will teach you what to say." (Exodus 4:11…12)

And just as God had faithfully promised to help Moses speak His words through the panic – and then commanded him to go – so He had with me.

I began to question why I hadn't read this passage in the weeks before sharing our testimony. Why I hadn't received that same reassurance *before* I got up on that stage. And I realised – I had to walk through that conversation with God myself.

I went further back in the passage, *before* God had reassured Moses of His help, and read as Moses threw his staff on the ground and it became a snake. Moses ran from it, seemingly afraid, but despite his fear – or maybe *because* of it – God instructed him to reach out his hand and pick up the snake. And in total trust, a still-fearful Moses obeyed. Before God promised to give him the words and help him to speak, Moses first had to step out in faith and – in his fear – pick up that snake.

Getting up on a public stage to speak my testimony of God's power and healing was my snake.

Since that day, God has guided and led me into more public speaking, each time more challenging than the one before. With Matt at our home church. With Matt at another church. Without Matt at a women's conference and other events. And then, in a full circle that only God can orchestrate, sharing my testimony publicly on-air at the very same radio station my panic attacks began at, fourteen years earlier.

Did I still feel incredibly nervous each time I spoke? Absolutely. But in obedience to God's prompting that final night in hospital – to not be silent about His healing works – I had to step out in faith. And then, just as He did with Moses, He taught me the words to say and helped me to speak them.

He took the trauma and pain of my time in hospital and used it to break a fourteen-year grip of fear, panic and shame.

All for His glory.

Chapter Twenty Seven

"You should write a book about what you went through". Words I heard over and again from many people in the months after coming home from hospital. From very early on I realised the interest in what had happened to me, the almost fascination that it provoked in people during a unique and emotional time. But the idea of writing a book about my experience was something I couldn't remotely comprehend. At that stage I couldn't remember any of the events leading up to the coma, I was still deeply traumatised by the days after coming off life support, and it would take many months to even begin to piece together some understanding of what had happened.

And yet... here I am. And here this book is. So what happened? Time happened. The proverbial healer of all wounds (along with bold prayer and an ECMO machine, as I can attest to!). It was around eighteen months after I came home from hospital – a year and a half of appointments, scans, conversations, memories, participation in medical research programs, shared public testimonies – that I felt the prompting to begin writing this book. I began the process with no idea of how it would look or what its purpose would be. I simply prayed and wrote.

I'm not one for leaning on cliches, but at times it truly has been an emotional rollercoaster to write. There have been many tears as memories return and moments are relived. There's the fear that comes from writing about a place of weakness and humility that feels incredibly vulnerable.

Around six months into the book I found myself in a very dark space every time I sat down to write. I often struggled to articulate my thoughts without being drawn back into the darkness and heaviness of the circumstances I was writing about. And then I contracted covid again in April 2024, the first time since the coma exactly two years earlier. Seeing the dark red positive line appear on the rapid antigen test again felt as sharp as a punch in the gut, as emotional memories instantly resurfaced and panic threatened to spill over. Despite committing my health, my anxieties, my life to God over and again over the past two years, we now realised this very moment had been hanging over us for so long – the waiting, the uncertainty, the what ifs. And so again we laid our fears at the feet of the One who is in control and, under the remote care of medical staff at Fiona Stanley Hospital, we felt a peaceful trust as to how the coming days would unfold. My body's response to the virus this time was completely different to the first, and I recovered strongly – at home, the chattering sounds of family life my healing soundtrack, with not an ECMO machine, hospital isolation room or PPE-clad doctor in sight.

Two weeks later I returned to my writing, and the shift in mindset was startlingly clear. I felt a sense of freedom, and the words now flowed from a heart and mind no longer inextricably tied in darkness to the situation I was writing about. I remembered the words of a kind nurse on the day I prepared to leave hospital, well-meaning in their intended reassurance: "Don't worry love, one day you'll forget all about this whole horrendous experience". And my response to her, honest and simple in my early understanding of God's healing power – "I truly pray I never do".

For I am forever changed by what happened – that I know with certainty. I seek to praise God for this every extra day I've been given. Healing is not always a straightforward process or, as a friend once said to me, "cut and dried and tied with a bow". It remains an ongoing journey of trust, of surrender, of weakness and strength, of accepting a peace that goes beyond my human understanding (Philippians 4:7). But I trust wholeheartedly in the purpose from the pain. His purpose from the pain, to accomplish what is now being done.

The hold of fear has been broken, and I'm no longer bound by the darkness.

In the morning came the light.

*For what we preach is not ourselves, but
Jesus Christ as Lord...
For God, who said "Let light shine out of
darkness", made his light shine in our hearts to
give us the light of the knowledge of God's glory
displayed in the face of Christ.*

(2 Corinthians 4: 5-6)

References

1. 'Way Maker' written and recorded by Sinach (Osinachi Okoro) in 2015. From the album *Way Maker (Live)*.

2. *I'm Not Crazy, I'm Just A Little Unwell* by Leigh Hatcher, Strand Publishing, 2005.

3. *Surviving Survival* by M. Little, C. Jordens, K. Paul and E. Sayers, Choice Books, Marrickville, 2001.

About the Author

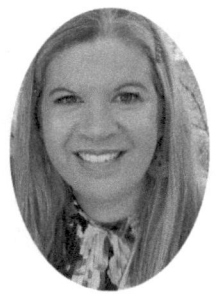

Abbey Spinelli is a wife and mother of two boys. Since graduating university, her varied professional roles over the years have included secondary school English and Drama teacher, magazine editor, features writer, broadcast journalist, news director, radio newsreader, education assistant and library officer – all of which have encouraged her love of words and storytelling! By far her most important and rewarding role, however, has been raising her two sons Jesaia and Coby with husband Matthew.

Abbey enjoys spending time with family and friends in nature, hiking in the forest and walking on the beach with her greyhound – thankfully, she lives in the beautiful southwest of Western Australia, so can do all three often! She's also very partial to eating Ferrero Rocher chocolate and reading autobiographies – ideally at the same time.

Connect with Abbey at https://inthemorningcamethelight.blogspot.com

www.ingramcontent.com/pod-product-compliance
Lightning Source LLC
Chambersburg PA
CBHW022055290426
44109CB00014B/1105